TRANQUILITY LOST

THE OCCUPATION OF TRANQUILLE AND BATTLE FOR COMMUNITY CARE IN BC

TRANQUILITY LOST

GARY STEEVES

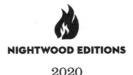

NIGHTWOOD EDITIONS

2020

Nightwood Editions
P.O. Box 1779
Gibsons, BC VON IVO
Canada
www.nightwoodeditions.com

COVER DESIGN: TopShelf Creative
TYPOGRAPHY: Shed Simas / Onça Design

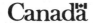

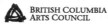

Nightwood Editions acknowledges the support of the Canada Council for the Arts, the Government of Canada, and the Province of British Columbia through the BC Arts Council.

This book has been produced on 100% post-consumer recycled, ancient-forest-free paper, processed chlorine-free and printed with vegetable-based dyes.

Printed and bound in Canada.

LIBRARY AND ARCHIVES CANADA CATALOGUING IN PUBLICATION
Title: Tranquility lost / by Gary Steeves.
Names: Steeves, Gary, author.
Identifiers: Canadiana (print) 20200213784 | Canadiana (ebook) 20200214810 |
    ISBN 9780889713864 (softcover) | ISBN 9780889713871 (ebook)
Subjects: LCSH: Intellectual disability facilities—British Columbia—Employees—History—20th
    century. | LCSH: Long-term care facilities—British Columbia—Employees—
    History—20th century. | LCSH: Mental health personnel—Employment—British
    Columbia—History—20th century. | LCSH: Collective bargaining—Health facilities—
    British Columbia—History—20th century. | LCSH: Intellectual disability facilities
    patients—British Columbia—History—20th century.
Classification: LCC RC448.B82 S74 2020 | DDC 331.89/041362230971109048—dc23

This book is dedicated with love to my wife Marina Horvath, who has put up with me for over forty years, through the events portrayed in this book, as well as the researching, organizing and writing.

CONTENTS

Foreword by Stephanie Smith   IX

Foreword by Cliff Andstein   XI

CHAPTER 1: Back in Business   1

CHAPTER 2: The Legislative Assault   22

CHAPTER 3: A Union Response   41

CHAPTER 4: From Dominance to Demise   57

CHAPTER 5: Running the Institution   75

CHAPTER 6: Legal Threats   89

CHAPTER 7: The Fear of Failure   104

CHAPTER 8: New Management Operations   120

CHAPTER 9: Songs, Poetry and Protest   137

CHAPTER 10: Negotiations and De-occupation   154

CHAPTER 11: It's About the Residents   173

EPILOGUE   189

Acknowledgements   203

Index   205

About the Author   211

STEPHANIE SMITH

I was one of those really annoying kids who would often say, "But that isn't fair!" though it turns out that fairness has proven to be one of the driving factors in my life. It's the reason why I became a union activist and it's the reason why the story of the occupation of Tranquille resonates so strongly with me. It was obvious that what was happening under the Bill Bennett government was not fair—it was not fair to the workers and it was not fair to the residents who lived at Tranquille.

When I joined the BCGEU in 1996, I became a member of the community social services component. This component came into existence ten years after Tranquille closed and includes the amazing people who support adults with developmental disabilities. It was those members who first told me what had occurred at Tranquille. The story of the occupation is a story of what happens when people who have long advocated and fought for others advocate and fight for themselves, and how those two things are inextricably inter-twined. It's about collective action, a common purpose and ultimately about triumph.

I am extremely proud to be the president of a union where the lessons learned from the collective action at Tranquille are baked into our DNA, where social justice combines with worker power to effect positive change. I'm grateful to Gary Steeves for telling this story and humbled to be a part of this project in some small way.

Stephanie Smith
President, BC Government and Service Employees' Union

CLIFF ANDSTEIN

"I n every Ministry, in every government office, in every crown corporation and in every public body, restraint measures will be taken."

With these words on July 7, 1983, while introducing his budget, Social Credit finance minister Hugh Curtis launched a neoliberal attack on the human, social, union and other rights of British Columbians. The twenty-six bills introduced that day broke the social contract between the government and people of British Columbia by bringing Reaganism and Thatcherism to the province. No sector or group, except for the corporations and businesspeople, escaped the attack. The poor, children, women, immigrants, unions, the disabled and the elderly saw their fundamental rights weakened or stripped in one of the most vicious right-wing attacks by a government since the Depression.

People of the province were in shock. Within days, protests were organized. Six thousand people attended a rally in Victoria organized by the BC Federation of Labour and the BC Government Employees' Union. The protests grew throughout July. Twenty-five thousand "massed in fury" according to the Victoria *Times Colonist* and within a few days, twenty thousand gathered in Vancouver. Virtually every community in the province saw protest marches or demonstrations against the government's legislation. While they were being organized, an unplanned event took place in Tranquille institution for people with intellectual and developmental issues.

As part of its restraint program, the government down-sized or closed institutions that provided services such as those delivered at Tranquille, or geriatric or mental health institutions. The move was cloaked in language suggesting these closures were to replace outdated institutions with contemporary community facilities and resources. The truth is the community resources simply did not exist. The BCGEU, which represented the majority of the workers at Tranquille, received an invitation in mid-July from the Ministry of Human Resources to attend a meeting to discuss "Tranquille." No further information was provided.

Gary Steeves attended this meeting and was shocked by the announcement that the ten-year plan for phasing out Tranquille by 1991 was now accelerated to 1984, just one year away. Additionally, the union was threatened with the removal of the collective agreement language that dealt with closures and redundancies. The ministry officials said they would invoke two of the pieces of legislation, Bills 2 and 3, which stripped the union's master agreement of those protections. The union representatives were stunned.

The meeting set off a chain of events that helped mobilize and inspire people around British Columbia as they began organizing to fight back against the government. Steeves flew to Kamloops to speak to BCGEU membership at II p.m. that night. Most stewards and local officers showed up along with many of the union members who worked at the institution. Steeves reported to the three hundred members on the details of the meeting earlier that day. The room became completely silent. He asked them, "Do you want to fight back?"

A member stood up and said loud and clear, "We have no choice!" The members in the room erupted into a loud standing ovation and within the hour, plans were made to occupy the institution and place it "under new management" beginning the following day: July 20, 1983. When the occupation of Tranquille was reported in the media later that day, it served as an inspiration to people all over the province that they could fight back. Support for the union and the workers in Tranquille came from all over Canada.

This book is a first-hand account in which Steeves takes us through what it means to occupy and administer a facility housing and serving some of the most vulnerable residents in the province. He begins with a discussion of the development of the healthcare system in British Columbia, the growth of public mental health institutions, the changing attitudes to treatment models and the move away from residential care institutions.

Tranquility Lost tells the story of the occupation and ongoing management of a mental health institution with 600 dedicated staff caring for the 325 residents. Steeves effectively captures the drama of those few weeks at Tranquille in 1983: the excitement of the workers, the anger at government and the commitment of the staff to the residents. This is a compelling story about what can be achieved when workers and their unions fight back against injustice and governments that use the coercive power of legislation.

Cliff Andstein
fomer collective bargaining and arbitration director,
BC Government and Service Employees' Union

CHAPTER ONE

BACK IN BUSINESS

T he proposal in 1983 by the Social Credit provincial government to close Tranquille School in Kamloops, BC, was nothing new. The Social Credit Party and government had adopted the stance that deinstitutionalization was a sound public policy goal. Furthermore, red-headed Socred icon and human resources minister Grace McCarthy had emerged as a leading proponent, primarily because the provincial institutions caring for people with developmental delays were in her ministry.

In the opinion of many observers, the Socreds' fixation with the goal was based on the cost savings government might realize from the closure of institutions. After a great deal of experience, I came to believe this about the Socreds, too. To them, the consideration of alternate care models for vulnerable British Columbians was secondary to saving money, if it was considered at all. The prospect of reducing the size of government and saving money was just too

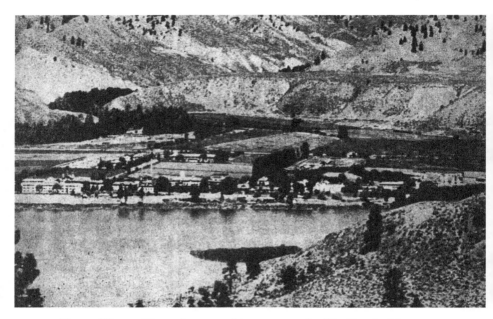

Photo of Tranquille on the cover of BCGEA magazine The Provincial,
April 1954. BCGEU Archives

enticing for Social Credit. Money, not human compassion, was the driving force behind McCarthy and the Social Credit government of Premier Bill Bennett.

The Tranquille Institution in Kamloops, BC was a supported residence for people with developmental disabilities. It had a long history of providing services in the Kamloops area and was a major part of the regional economy. Prior to providing education and training to persons with intellectual challenges, it served as a tuberculosis sanatorium. Tranquille was located just outside Kamloops on high plains above the Tranquille River. In 1983, it had about 600 full- and part-time staff caring for about 325 residents. The Ministry of Human Resources operated the institution with the intention of educating and training people with developmental disabilities to prepare them for living in the community. Between the end of the 1950s and the early 1980s, 460 developmentally delayed residents had been placed from Tranquille into community-living situations. As residents with mild and moderate developmental disabilities successfully transitioned into the community, Tranquille's resident population increasingly became people with more profound developmental disabilities. The ministry's mission and the work of its staff to facilitate community living placement became increasingly more difficult.

The institution was physically huge with forty buildings, its own fire department, powerhouse, industrial laundry, maintenance shops, a canteen, stores and a substantial farm. The farm had 300 acres under irrigation, 150 acres of natural hay meadows, 300 acres of grazing meadows and 13,400 acres of range land. These lands facilitated the raising of 160 head of beef cattle including 50 head of young stock, 75 bulls and 30 steers, 75 Holstein milking cows, 150 breeding cows and 500 hogs. All feeds except grain were grown on the farm. The Tranquille Farm was operated by the provincial Ministry of Agriculture and supported Tranquille's dietary department, which produced sixty-five thousand meals monthly. It also provided a host of training and educational opportunities for residents.

Regardless of the complexities of the institution and the challenges and successes of the past decades, the late 1970s and early 1980s saw the growth of a movement toward deinstitutionalization. Advocates effectively made the argument that people with special needs deserved community-based care, referring to institutional care as "human warehousing" and "old-fashioned and inhumane." Their vision of community-based care saw a no less expensive care model. Advocates for community care wanted extensive community-based services and support systems.

The provincial government's goal to reduce per capita expenditures was not part of the advocates' agenda. But this fundamental disagreement was set aside, at least temporarily, as the advocates embraced the Social Credit's deinstitutionalization policy platform. After all, the government had successfully closed the Skeenaview institution in Terrace and Dellview in Vernon. The advocates were comforted by this track record and put aside their differences over funding as government proposed the closure of all institutions for people with developmental disabilities.

BC's Social Credit Party came into BC electoral politics in the 1949 BC general election. It ran as the BC Social Credit League (BCSCL) and put forth nine candidates. They received only 3,072 votes total for the province and did not elect any members to the legislative assembly.

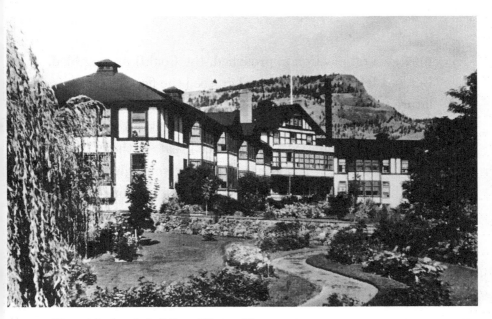

The original main building at Tranquille. BCGEU Archives

The 1949 election was dominated by what was known as the Coalition, a group of Liberal and Conservative MLAs including W.A.C. Bennett, the Progressive Conservative MLA for South Okanagan. The Coalition took 61.35 percent of the provincial popular vote and Bennett won his constituency with 58.4 percent of the votes cast. The Official Opposition, the Co-operative Commonwealth Federation (CCF), won 35.1 percent of the provincial vote but only seven seats in the legislature. The pro-business, centre-right coalition had kept the leftist CCF at bay for another electoral term.

Despite their 1949 electoral success, the Coalition grew increasingly unpopular over the next three years. As the

1952 general election approached, the Coalition crumbled. Bennett left the Coalition and crossed the floor of the legislature to join the new Social Credit Party (BCSCL). Under a new preferential voting system intended to keep out the CCF, Social Credit went on to win nineteen seats in the 1952 general election. The Official Opposition CCF won eighteen seats and the highest popular vote (34.3 percent) among the parties. The Liberal and Conservative parties won six and four seats respectively and a minority Social Credit government headed by W.A.C. Bennett took office.

The minority Social Credit government did not last the year and British Columbians found themselves back at the polls on June 9, 1953. With the preferential voting system in place again, the final results gave W.A.C. a healthy majority. With less than half the popular vote (45.5 percent), Social Credit won a solid majority of twenty-eight seats in the forty-three-seat legislature. Bennett then brought back first-past-the-post voting and didn't look back.

Following 1952, W.A.C. Bennett would govern as BC premier for twenty years. W.A.C.'s populist approach on many issues had built a loyal base for his Social Credit Party. The polarized world of BC politics, due mainly to the collapse of the provincial Liberal and Conservative parties, persisted through the 1950s and 1960s. And the steady economic growth of the period suffered only a temporary setback in the late 1950s. Bennett's government cemented its reputation as a pro-business, socially conservative group by responding to the recession in typical right-wing fashion. It cut spending, eliminated hundreds of public employees' jobs and slashed welfare payments to the poor.

By 1965, the Bennett government had set a record for the longest continuous government in office by a BC political party. Its 1966 re-election was a walk in the park as Social Credit captured thirty-three of the fifty-five seats in the provincial legislature. The opposition NDP elected sixteen MLAs. Social Credit's success as a provincial government continued through the 1969 election, when it recorded the highest share of the popular vote in BC history with 46.79 percent. The 1969 election saw the opposition NDP reduced to twelve seats. NDP Leader Tom Berger went down to personal defeat in his riding of Vancouver-Burrard. Few could foresee any slippage in the Social Credit's grip on power.

Social Credit enjoyed a thriving BC economy fuelled by logging and mining. The coastal forests of Douglas fir, western cedar, balsam fir, hemlock and Sitka spruce provided an abundance of fibre in the mild wet climate, supporting an industry unconcerned with environmental issues. The interior forest industry had lodgepole pine, ponderosa pine and aspen in addition to the coastal species. Accessing markets with timber and mineral products, however, required infrastructure. WAC Bennett did not hesitate to address industry's needs. His prompt attention to the needs of industry stood in stark contrast to his response to the poor and underprivileged. Bennett saw government's role as initiating ambitious projects such as road building and power megaprojects. Social safety nets were not a priority for him but he made sure the rail line to northeast BC was completed. He made sure the north and the central interior was connected to the more heavily populated southwest corner of the province. The Kelowna hardware merchant guided BC along the road to economic expansion.

The critique that the CCF/NDP opposition levied at Social Credit was mainly centred on three themes. First, BC resources were being given away for a song. Resource royalty revenue lagged far behind what was being collected by governments in other jurisdictions and this lost revenue meant British Columbians were being ripped off. Second, the NDP said, the BC resource revenue rip-off meant the government did not have the financial ability to address urgent social priorities of the people. Bennett did not regard social programs as important. Health and social service program reforms were ignored by Bennett as he channelled money back into the industries that supported his vision of the provincial economy.

The third criticism was focused on the multitude of societal problems created by an inadequate social safety net in the province. Programs for the vulnerable and assistance for those in need were either minimally funded or non-existent. Bennett appeared oblivious to the needs of the poor or the criticism of his government's attitude toward them. With an ever-expanding provincial economy, BC's social safety net trailed far behind other Canadian provinces and developed economies around the world. Even as corporate profits increased, the province made little effort to deal with inadequate hospital facilities, poor mental health services, and incompetent or non-existent care for the elderly.

As successive Bennett governments rolled through the 1960s, the criticism became sharper and more specific. BC needed to be modernized, critics said. A small example was the legislature's lack of Hansard Services. No record of what the representatives of the people had said or were saying was available to the public. But Hansard, it was argued, costs money and was an intrusion into the unrestricted debate of the legislature. By the 1972 election, BC's Socreds had governed for twenty years and were being characterized as old and tired. BC's NDP compared the BC shortcomings with the success of Saskatchewan's NDP government. In Saskatchewan, handsome resource royalties were collected, automobile insurance was more cheaply offered by a Crown corporation and social programs treated people more adequately. Bennett, they said, was out of touch. Some people in BC noted the irony of Bennett's criticism of the NDP as socialist hordes who wanted to nationalize private industry. Bennett, in his zeal to open up the interior and the north and supply industry with reliable power as well as provide the province with a stable transportation grid, had nationalized BC Electric to create BC Hydro; nationalized Black Ball Ferries to create the BC Ferry Corp.; and drove BC

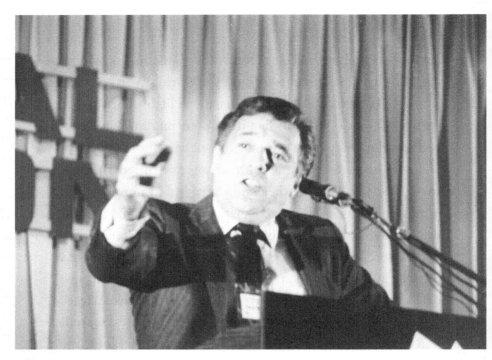

Dave Barrett, BC premier 1972–75 and leader of the opposition 1975–84.

Rail to the far reaches of the Peace River country. Bennett may have been out of touch with the people, but he was in sync with the industrial leaders who could deliver for him. Just don't be poor, old, sick or infirm.

The unexpected 1972 victory of Dave Barrett and the New Democrats has been well chronicled by Geoff Meggs and Rod Mickleburgh in their excellent book *The Art of the Impossible: Dave Barrett and the NDP in Power 1972–1975.* Government modernization and enhancement of human services as well as the establishment of public institutions like the Agricultural Land Commission, the Insurance Corporation of BC and the Human Rights Commission remain hallmarks of the Barrett government. The advancement of services to women in particular resulted in the development of rape relief centres, women's health collectives, daycares and the guaranteed minimum income (Mincome) for those over sixty.

In total, the Barrett government had enacted a total 367 pieces of legislation, about two per week while in office. The 1975 provincial election campaign, however, took BC back in a more familiar direction. In 1972, the NDP had 39.6 percent of the provincial popular vote compared to Social Credit's 31.2 percent. In 1975, the NDP retained its share of the popular vote, receiving 39.1 percent and received a few more actual votes than they had received in 1972. But Social Credit got 49.3 percent of the popular vote as the Liberal and Conservative vote collapsed.

The NDP election slogan in '75 was "People Matter More." New premier-elect Bill Bennett mocked the slogan on election night, saying that "people, not glib slogans, won the election," but his government was not as interested in people as it was in supporting corporate profitability. Dave Barrett's "free drugs for seniors" philosophy was quickly vanquished. Bennett immediately assisted the mining and forest industries by dismantling the Mineral Royalties Act and addressing industry concerns about timber royalties.

Liberal Leader Gordon Gibson described the demise of his Liberal Party and the arrival of the new Socred government as "a kind of tidal wave of support for the political right." Social Credit was back in business. By the 1980s, Bill Bennett had "greased every skid" to get industry into the improved profit column. Like his father, Bill Bennett had a love affair with megaprojects. The Coquihalla Highway, BC Place Stadium, the Vancouver Trade and Convention Centre and the Lower Mainland's Skytrain are all examples of the government's belief that bigger was better. Just don't be poor, old or sick. Bennett balanced the government's generosity to corporations with cuts to government spending on social programs and restraint on public service and teacher salaries.

Bennett's megaproject spending (such as one billion tax dollars on the development of Northeast Coal) required a broad public sector restraint program. Extensive cutbacks to government services and the outright elimination of some government programs echoed the Social Credit mantra that government was bad and private capital was good. Government employees paid an immediate price for the government's philosophical beliefs. Government programs, no matter how sparse, were considered generous by Social Credit standards. The health and social service ministries were not spared in the restraint mentality and the provincial institutions they operated continued to struggle from restraints placed on human and capital investment.

In a December 16, 1982 cabinet meeting, ministers reviewed a "Staff Review of Restraint" which cited the 5 percent savings highways had realized due to privatization and the loss of seven hundred employees. It projected further savings as each ministry reduced staff by 250 to 500 employees. But the deputy minister of human resources wrote to cabinet advising of the peculiar circumstances of MHR institutions like Tranquille. The memo said, "A major reduction in the staff in the institutions at this time would jeopardize the overall plan toward decentralized care of people with intellectual challenges. Therefore, the ministry is proposing only a 12 percent cutback at this time."

All that would change in the near future. Shortly after Bennett's May 5, 1983 election victory, he convened a cabinet and caucus retreat in the Okanagan to discuss the program his newly re-elected government should present to British Columbians. The featured speaker was a senior advisor to Margaret Thatcher, and the favourite whipping boys for the meeting were public institutions, unions and social programs. Reducing the size and scope of government was the overriding issue. The Fraser Institute provided facilitators for the critical discussions about the future of BC.

The Bennett government, over successive terms, became even more heavily influenced by the Fraser Institute. The Institute was a creation of the leadership of BC's largest corporations during the term of the 1972–75 NDP government and it ensured that Social Credit had an unending supply of neoliberal research and propaganda material. The conservative economic theories espoused by Milton Friedman were always front of mind as Bennett watched Thatcher and Reagan redefine their countries' economic and social values. Featuring massive tax cuts to the rich, the crushing of trade unions, deregulation, and privatization of public services, the road map espoused by the Fraser Institute captivated Social Credit. Cabinet ministers had already involved themselves in cabinet-level discussions about the nature of the provincial economy and the service demands on government. A January 26, 1982 cabinet meeting discussed a Garde Gardom memo on "Emerging Issues in Social Services" citing an "aging population, unemployment [and] native persons" as three reasons why social service costs needed to be addressed. By the November 25, 1982 cabinet meeting, ministers were ready to make some decisions based on their deliberations over the previous year. Government wanted economic reform and a reduction of the public service.

On November 25, 1982, cabinet accepted and supported the report on the "Accelerated Program of Government Activity in the Forest, Mining and Transportation Sectors 1982/83." This program was a major part of the government's economic recovery and job creation program. It channelled large amounts of money to industry and the formal, legal mechanism to provide taxpayer support to good old free enterprise and its market economy. Apparently, the cabinet believed that government could be a flow-through agency, redirecting tax dollars to private industry without a bureaucratic structure to waste money on.

At the same meeting, ministers approved "Contingency Vote 40, Reallocation of Funds," which required the redirection of any savings from the Compensation Stabilization Program (CSP) in the public sector "to these economic recovery/job creation measures." Simultaneously the cabinet shamelessly decided to "reduce government grants by April 1, 1983" by "capping" MHR transfers at 20 percent. The CSP was the government's chosen method to restrain wages in the broader public sector and Contingency Vote 40 made it impossible to reallocate those funds to public service programs such as community resources for Tranquille residents. Bennett was single-minded in his belief that the private sector's major employers were to be supported at all cost.

Cabinet documents show that while the government was bailing out company after company (a dam upgrade for Tech Cominco, road maintenance for Granduc Mining, bankruptcy bailout for the Whistler Village Land Co. to name a few), education, health and social service expenditures were being restrained and public service expenditures cut. One January 1983 cabinet document looking at MHR expenditures said, "Other specialized services to be terminated are the post-partum counselling team, the Medical Clinic, in-home services and family and child assessment teams." It was all about money for Social Credit and they knew exactly what they were doing. Although their specific measures did not always jive with the principles of free enterprise, the government's public pronouncements tried to suggest otherwise.

The size of government was always a political measure used by Social Credit and they deliberately and vigorously pursued reductions. A February 22, 1983 memo from the assistant deputy minister of intergovernmental relations to the secretary to the cabinet committee on social services explained Treasury Board Order 57 saying, "the policy is established to cover two situations... forced relocation and redundancy." The memo noted that, "the policy allows alternative work at the present location or termination with severance pay or early retirement where the employee meets the eligibility criteria." To the cabinet, that was a cost that needed to be brought under control.

The Social Credit caucus discussion took place within the paradigm of an unswerving belief that competition is the defining characteristic of human relations. As British investigative journalist and author George Monbiot has explained, "Democratic choices were best exercised by buying and selling, a process that rewards merit and punishes inefficiency." But the government did not consistently act that way. Perhaps the most controversial tenet of the neoliberal philosophy was that "the Market" was the very best way to organize modern society. That this system would produce winners and losers was only natural because the market would make sure everyone got what they deserved. Did that mean that if you were poor, you deserved to have nothing to eat? Yes! said the pro-market philosophy. The poor were economic losers and Bennett, by his own admission, thought those who disagreed with him were "bad British Columbians." His government eagerly considered a radical program to make the market the dominant decision-maker in BC.

The changes that would have to be made were to be laid out in the July 1983 budget and its accompanying legislation. The drastic nature of the legislative program and budget came in sharp contrast to the January 27, 1983 presentation to cabinet by the BC Chamber of Commerce. The Chamber expressed its optimism about the economic recovery that had started and made "practical suggestions" to the government about the things they saw as problems. They asked for lower hydro rates, prevention of ferry strikes, property tax relief and money for the tourism industry. The Chamber encouraged the continuation of the government's involvement in primary industries such as forestry and mining and wanted secondary picketing outlawed. And that was it.

The MLAs, however, talked about advocacy and the need to control "special-interest groups." According to senior staff of the day, the Bennett cabinet wanted their opposition crushed. Advocacy groups and organizations, big and small, needed to be stifled if Social Credit's reforms were to be achieved. The Social Credit caucus knew the BC Government Employees' Union (BCGEU) and other unions would

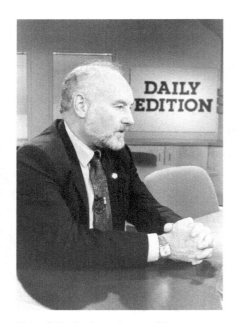

John Shields, first vice-president of the BCGEU, in 1983. BCGEU Archives

oppose the budget and labour legislation like Bills 2 and 3 and the Employment Standards Act amendments. The caucus agreed that curtailing union power was critical to reducing the size and cost of government. The Social Credit caucus also knew the BCGEU and other labour organizations were the best organized and best funded of all the special interest organizations to oppose the 1983 budget and its accompanying legislation. Bills 2 and 3 would stifle the BCGEU, and Bill 2 would eliminate its power to fight the government. The legislation would give the government the tools it needed to curtail the strength of the BCGEU opposition.

On the day the legislation was tabled, still a long way from becoming law, the government began terminating public sector employees. The Socreds fired the two executive vice-presidents of the BCGEU from their provincial government jobs—John Shields and Diane Wood. On July 7, they sent letters to hundreds of employees, the text of which had been approved by cabinet. The letter to the human rights branch employees, signed by acting deputy minister Isabel A. Kelly, said, "This is to advise you that as a result of legislation tabled today, the Human Rights Branch and Commission will be eliminated. As a result of this legislation, and in anticipation of the changes, we are cutting back on staff and your position has become redundant." Did the government really think British Columbians would just roll over with compliance?

The government completely miscalculated the motivating effect the legislation and the termination

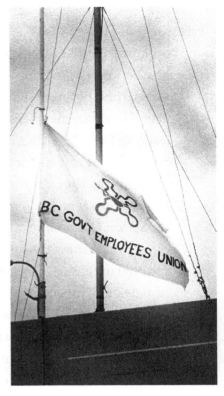

BCGEU flag at Tranquille.

BCGEU Archives

letters had on BCGEU members. Union membership acted as if they had been pinched in the rear end. Action broke out in most of the BCGEU's major locals. At times, it all felt like bewildering chaos as union headquarters tried to keep up with developments in various areas of the province. What government misunderstood completely was the ability of the union movement to come together with community organizations large and small, effectively opposing the offensive actions of government. There were thousands of small steps that defined the resistance to the government's agenda. BCGEU members and community allies worked tirelessly in this regard but in the sunny Okanagan in June, the Social Credit caucus thought they had it all figured out.

Cabinet thought the provincial unemployment rate of about 15 percent (20 percent in Kamloops) called for drastic action. Economic research over the next thirty-plus years would show that neoliberal conservative approaches resulted in significantly lower economic growth rates and an expansion of inequality in both income and wealth. Laissez-faire liberalism had revealed real problems in Europe in the last century but, not surprisingly, the very rich were the real beneficiaries of these right-wing policies.

Social Credit's long journey from the post-war years to the early eighties was marked by an evolution from a W.A.C.-led populist, pro-business government to a solid right-wing party with neoliberal economic and social policy. By 1983, they were completely wrapped in the cloak of Milton Friedman and Margaret Thatcher, and prepared to see what a majority government could do in BC. In 1983, Bill Bennett was riding high on a newly elected majority government with a well-defined political program and influential right-wing allies in the business and academic worlds. Cabinet records from 1982 through to Bennett's departure in 1986 show his government providing a steady stream of grants, rebates, forgivable loans and special tax measures for private companies and business organizations.

While ordinary taxpayers subsidized corporate life, the loss of union rights, human rights, tenants' rights and other advocacy tools would be their reward. Bennett believed a complete transformation was entirely within his grasp, with only the passage of a few pieces of legislation standing between the current recession and economic prosperity. At least that is what Bennett and his caucus said publicly as they proceeded to the legislature on July 7 to tell British Columbians what was good for them. But Tranquille workers did not think much of the budget and its legislative package. The Social Credit philosophy and budget legislation provided the backdrop for a dramatic occupation in Kamloops and unprecedented militancy from Tranquille and other BC workers.

CHAPTER TWO

THE LEGISLATIVE ASSAULT

B ill Bennett's confidence was on full display when the legislature opened on June 23, 1983 and did not diminish as Finance Minister Hugh Curtis rose in the legislature shortly after 2 p.m. on Thursday, July 7, 1983 "to present the Government of British Columbia budget for the fiscal year ending March 31, 1984." It was an annual event where government boasted of its achievements and revealed grand plans for the future. The opposition, for its part, attempted to find as many flaws as possible with the government's performance and criticize the government's plans. Opposition criticism that year was focused on the finance minister in particular.

Curtis began by stating that he remained committed to a set of four philosophical principles. None seemed particularly philosophical, but he may have felt the need to sound reasoned and thoughtful. The minister's approach might seem obvious later. Curtis outlined his "unalterable dedication to the financial accountability of government to the people." Next, he made a vague pronouncement of being committed to financial responsibility in case anyone thought finance ministers may be committed to irresponsibility. His third commitment was to the principle of fairness. And his fourth and final so-called

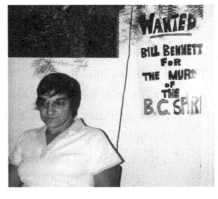

Signs were everywhere during the occupation including this "wanted" poster for Bill Bennett. Gary Steeves

principle was a commitment "to a government role in the economy which supports private initiative, which provides permanent and rewarding jobs and which builds a secure and prosperous economic future."

The first three so-called principles—financial accountability, financial responsibility, and fairness—were hardly new or earth-shattering. BC laws generally provided for these notions of public responsibility; Curtis was really reiterating practical considerations for any finance minister. The three were more competency indicators than philosophical debating points. The fourth principle, however, was different. It was more like the Social Credit neoliberal mantra to justify the coming budget as well as previous cabinet decisions like Vote 40. This so-called "principle" was the one that set the direction for the Bill Bennett government and its intention to reshape BC in the image of Margaret Thatcher and Ronald Reagan. Curtis was trying to establish a rationale for setting aside the public good and government responsibility for British Columbians in favour of corporate welfare and the corporate good as defined by capital markets and Social Credit friends.

Curtis outlined his analysis of the provincial economy since the 1960s. He noted the faltering prosperity and "economic crisis of the past two years." Recovery, he said, should not and cannot be taken for granted as the problems BC faced today "originated in the social and economic fabric woven through at least two decades of prosperity and social reform." Curtis was advancing an astonishing twist of logic. He was asserting that the international recession impacting BC was caused by the "prosperity and social reform" advanced by previous BC governments. Hard to believe that a finance minister would make such an argument but Hansard caught it all. According to the finance minister, we were all too prosperous and living too high on the hog while human rights interfered with the entrepreneurial spirit.

Curtis apparently saw no need to notify MLAs that government would, later that day, table its best efforts to eliminate those pesky job-killing social reforms. In detailed and blunt language, he outlined the problem with governments using social or environmental programs to get in the way of private-sector initiative and growth. According to Curtis, public sector employment was a problem in BC and in Canada. Borrowing to finance prosperity was even more problematic, he said, because interest rates "reached levels in excess of 20 percent." This was especially "devastating" for BC, argued Curtis, because the 1982 Social Credit budget had overestimated revenue by almost $1 billion ($872 million to be precise). The overestimation was not slight, and the reason for this gross overestimation seemed obvious to the opposition. Social Credit wanted to campaign for the May 1983 general election on a balanced budget and needed to overestimate revenue to do so.

The finance minister was lengthy and deliberate in outlining his view of the economic issues facing BC. He noted the provincial gross domestic product "declined by some 7 percent in 1982 compared to a 4.4 percent decline nationally." Over 200,000 British Columbia workers were unemployed in the winter of 1982–83 with some 162,000 BC workers on UIC benefits. This level of economic displacement had substantially increased income assistance payments which further strained provincial finances. He did not mention the record number of working people trying to pay their mortgage with a 21-percent interest rate and he did not dwell on the budget's provision for closing Tranquille. Social Credit MLAs applauded his performance.

Opposition finance critic Dave Stupich was a seasoned debater and veteran counterpuncher. Replying to the finance minister's budget speech on July 8, Stupich was precise in his criticism of the budget: "Never in the history of the province of British Columbia have revenues been overestimated anything in the remote vicinity of the $872 million of the year just concluded." Stupich questioned the competency of the minister and his advisors as he continued his rebuttal of the Curtis record. How could any competent administration overestimate revenue by almost a billion dollars in one year? This, of course, was at a time when a million dollars was a big-ticket item in a provincial budget. Stupich continued by stating, "On April 5, 1982, the minister of finance had the gall to issue a statement under his name that he had produced an operating budget balanced by revenues. Figures released with the budget yesterday prove the utter falsehood that was presented to the people of British Columbia by the minister of finance on April 5." Stupich summed up his observations of the budget and those of many observers when he said, "We should all understand the budget to be a manipulation of an election promise." Curtis had said, "It is time to strive for more with less," but MLA Stupich mocked the budget, its accuracy and its validity as anything other than a Social Credit fantasy.

The Official Opposition continued to participate in the legislature's budget debate, probing various areas including issues raised in the election campaign just months before. Stupich pointed out that during the April–May 1983 election campaign, "the premier made vague references to continued restraint. It is also true that the Social Credit Party promised a total of $1.474 billion in new spending." The contradictions and manipulations in the budget presentation were debated at length and laid before the public for full consideration. Stupich had done his job as finance critic but the government seemed unmoved by fact or passion. They brushed aside the embarrassing truth of revenue deception and political double-talk and ended debate with the adoption of Bill 10 Supply Act (No. 1) 1983. The government had used its majority to approve a total budget of $6.043 billion for 1983–84. Nowhere in that vast sum of money was there any funds allocated for community-based support services for people with developmental disabilities.

The government forged ahead. Late in the afternoon of July 7 after Minister Curtis had completed his speech, the government tabled twenty-five additional pieces of legislation which drew intense legislative scrutiny. The world exploded as the scope and extent of the proposed legislation was revealed. Subsequent legislative debate and private analysis intensified public concern over the government's direction. The budget bills were a jolt to civil society. They covered virtually every aspect of public sector operation. They tinkered with taxation policy and began the tax shift away from private corporations and onto individual taxpayers. The proposed legislation included Bills 2 and 3, which alarmed the BCGEU to its core.

Bill 2 was formally called the Public Service Labour Relations Amendment Act. It would strip public sector collective agreements of protections and benefits for any worker in that bargaining unit and prohibit negotiations of such benefits in the future. For Tranquille workers, the bill meant they would lose layoff and recall protection, severance pay, job placement rights and a host of other benefits once their BCGEU collective agreements expired on October 31, 1983. It was a stunning piece of legislation that BCGEU analysts concluded would be the end of bona fide collective bargaining in the public sector.

Bill 3 was even more stunning, if that was possible. Called the Public Sector Restraint Act, it proposed to give government and government agencies, boards and commissions (in effect all public sector employers including local governments and school boards) the right to fire any employee without cause and for any reason, including no reason at all. Its application to teachers, hospital workers, school board employees, direct government employees, municipal employees, Crown corporation employees and more was almost beyond comprehension. Polling showed that over two-thirds of the BC public thought the government was wrong to propose the right to fire workers without cause. The measure rubbed the vast majority of British Columbians the wrong way and became one of the loudest protest points in the province-wide Operation Solidarity protest.

As early as the day the legislation was tabled, the telex machine at BCGEU headquarters in Burnaby began spewing copies of termination letters, or notice of termination

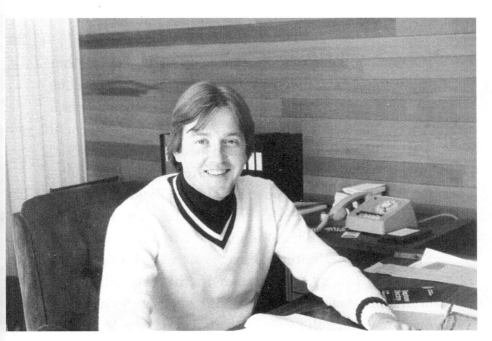

Gary Steeves, newly hired research officer for the BCGEU, in 1979.

BCGEU Archives

letters, sent to BCGEU members. I was astonished as the letters came. I knew almost all of the members the letters were addressed to: most were union activists, shop stewards, or local union executive members. I remember the feeling of astonishment at the government for arrogantly acting on a mere proposal before the legislature. And the upheaval and stress it caused in people's lives was reflected in the phone calls our union staff was receiving.

There was a host of other proposed legislation including Bill 18, the Pension (Public Service) Amendment Act; Bill 11, the Compensation Stabilization Act; Bill 25, the Harbour Board Repeal Act; Bill 21, the Crown Corporation Reporting Repeal Act; Bill 8, the Alcohol and Drug Commission Repeal Act; Bill 24, the Medical Services Act; Bill 5, the Residential Tenancy Act; Bill 16, the Employment Development Act; Bill 14, the Gasoline (Coloured) Tax Amendment Act; Bill 15, the Social Service Tax Amendment Act; Bill 13, the Tobacco Tax Act 1983; Bill 28, the Provincial Treasury Financing Amendment Act; Bill 4, the Income Tax Amendment Act; Bill 17, the Misc. Statutes (Finance Measures) Amendment Act 1983; Bill 27, the Human Rights Act; Bill 9, the Municipal Amendment Act; Bill 22, the Assessment Amendment Act; Bill 7, the Property Tax Reform Act; Bill 26, the Employment Standards Amendment Act; Bill 20, the College and Institutes Amendment Act; Bill 19, the Institute of Technology Amendment Act; and Bill 6, the Education (Interim) Finance Amendment Act 1983. None of it appeared particularly pro-worker.

The Operation Solidarity (Op Sol) movement was created by the BC Federation of Labour after the government tabled its twenty-six pieces of legislation on July 7. I briefed the Federation's Public Sector Committee on the afternoon of July 8 on the proposed legislation. The Collective Bargaining and Arbitration Department staff of the BCGEU had analyzed the bills and BCGEU Director Jack Adams, chair of the Fed's Public Sector Committee, had requested the briefing. The committee developed a strategy to fight the government, which was supported by the Fed through funding of the Op Sol movement. A full strategy eventually included a work stoppage schedule and a general strike of all BC Fed–affiliated unions. General strikes are more common in European countries and quite uncommon in North America. Needless to say, the Fed's plan of attack on the government's legislation generated immense media interest.

The legislative landslide caught almost everyone's attention. The Vancouver bureau of the *Globe and Mail* carried a two-page spread headlined, "Bennett's hard line: The 26 bills at centre of storm." If Bills 2 and 3 were not a strident enough attack on the labour movement, Bennett proposed Bill 27 to abolish the Human Rights Commission and the Human Rights branch of government. It unceremoniously closed hundreds of complaint case files and had security personnel confiscate office keys and escort employees out of their places of employment. On camera, it looked more like a military coup than the smooth operation of a British parliamentary democracy. In the Social Credit mind, tabling the legislation was as good as it being adopted. If Bills 2, 3, 26 and 27 did not catch a broad cross-section of the public's attention, the proposed phasing out of the provincial residential tenancy branch and the cancellation of assistance to tenants under Bill 5 had a chilling effect on a larger portion of BC citizens. And although one could use the legislative package to create an ever-growing list of aggrieved citizens, Bennett's government did not seem to care.

The spate of legislation tabled on July 7, 1983 was intended to meet the fundamental objectives for the Bennett government. Social Credit wanted to eliminate or reduce benefits and rights enjoyed by the people of BC. The legislative package would reduce government costs and improve private sector efficiency, they said. It shifted the cost of government onto individual taxpayers and away from private-sector businesses. So much for Curtis' principle of "fairness" as Canadians already bore two-thirds of the tax burden compared with corporations.

The finance minister had insisted in his July 7 speech to the legislature that "government had grown too large." To address that situation, Curtis explained in some detail how government was approaching its staffing issues. "From a base of 47,000 FTE [full-time equivalent] staff... authorized in April, 1982, staff reduction plans have brought government ministries down substantially." "The budget for 1983–84," he said, "will provide funding for 39,965 FTE staff, with further reductions planned for 1984–85." He gave as examples the BC Building Corporation, which would be cut by 10 percent, and the government vehicle fleet-management staff, which would be reduced by 20 percent.

Social Credit assumed that tabling the proposed legislation in the legislature meant only the formality of adoption remained. Again, they underestimated the strength of the opposition from the New Democratic Party's MLAs. The government response to the vigorous opposition to the budget

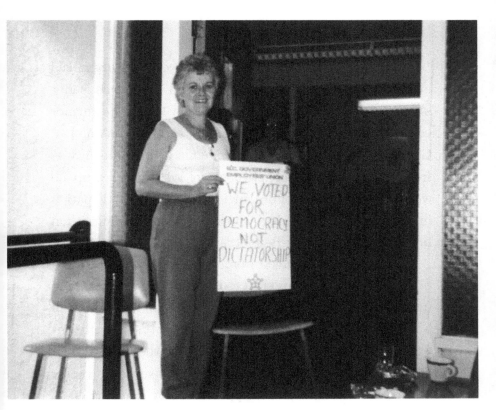

Denise Lietchfield, healthcare worker and key contributor to the phoning, scheduling and rostering committee. Gary Steeves

and the accompanying bills was to go to twenty-four-hour-a-day legislative sittings. The extended sittings and the use of closure would force their budget and the proposed legislation through the legislature more quickly. The use of the more draconian parliamentary closure would stifle debate and open the government to further criticism and accusations of undemocratic and dictatorial behaviour.

The opposition in the legislature would be organized and led by NDP leader Dave Barrett and his caucus leadership team. In a caucus full of veteran MLAs and former cabinet ministers, Barrett appointed a young MLA named Gordon Hanson as Opposition caucus whip. Hanson was from the two-member constituency of Victoria. As whip, he would be responsible for organizing the caucus participation in the round-the-clock, legislation-by-exhaustion marathon brought on by Premier Bennett's Socreds.

Hanson had received his master's degree in anthropology from the University of British Columbia and immediately went to work in the provincial museum in Victoria in the early seventies. Dave Barrett's government was in power and Hanson socialized with NDP political staffers including government caucus research director Mark Holtby. Hanson was approached by a government staffperson about the possibility of going to work in the office of Minister of Consumer Services Phyllis Young. Hanson applied for and was given a leave of absence (LOA) from his position at the museum, then went to work as ministerial assistant to Young for only a few months before Barrett dissolved the legislature and called the 1975 provincial election.

The timing of the 1975 election call has always raised controversy in NDP circles as the Barrett administration had nearly two years left in their legislative mandate. Hanson recalls a story that circulated among legislative staffers. Barrett had asked Provincial Secretary Ernie Hall if he could think of one reason why they should not drop the writ and go to the polls. Hall thought for a second and said, "I can think of fifty-eight thousand reasons." (The salary of a cabinet minister was $58,000 at the time.)

The legislature was dissolved on November 3, 1975, and Hanson sought and won the NDP nomination in the two-member constituency of Victoria. His running mate Charles Barber was a popular Victoria social activist and musician. On election day, Social Credit's Sam Bawlf topped the polls with Barber finishing second, just 498 votes behind. Hanson was third, 675 votes behind Barber. With Bawlf and Barber off to the legislature, Hanson was off to the unemployment line. Assistant provincial secretary and deputy to the premier Lawrie Wallace called Hanson to say he was too political to return to the museum. With no job and a marital breakup at hand, Hanson phoned his friend Cliff Andstein, BCGEU assistant general secretary. A short time later he was hired by the BCGEU to a job in the union's Burnaby headquarters. Hanson had been active in the union before taking his LOA from the museum. He had served in various capacities including chairperson of the Victoria local of the scientific component, chair of the province-wide scientific component executive and as a member of the union's provincial executive.

After two years in Burnaby working as a BCGEU staff representative, Hanson was transferred to the BCGEU's area office in Victoria. He re-engaged with local politics and was elected president of the Victoria NDP Constituency Association. As the 1979 provincial election approached, Hanson was again nominated with Charles Barber to contest the upcoming general election. He and Barber were successful in the two-member riding, with Hanson finishing three thousand votes ahead of Bawlf. The provincial results, although close, gave the NDP twenty-six seats in the legislature, five fewer than Social Credit, with an almost even split in the provincial popular vote. Hanson remained in the legislature, easily winning re-election in 1983. He and running mate Robin Blencoe beat their Socred challengers by more than seven thousand votes. Hanson's caucus leadership role in the Thirty-third Parliament of BC gave him a front-row seat to Premier Bennett's attempt to reshape BC through twenty-four-hour sittings of "legislation by exhaustion."

The Social Credit budget and spate of legislative bills were stark contrasts to the election outcome on May 5, 1983. Polling during that campaign periodically showed the NDP as a possible winner but on election day, the over 646,000 NDP votes were 2 percent short of the almost 678,000 Social Credit ballots. The NDP candidates in the '83 election represented an earlier generation of high-profile, solidly social democratic Party stalwarts like Frank Howard, Alex Macdonald, Dave Stupich and a handful of holdovers from Barrett's 1972 cabinet. And to make life more interesting,

Barrett announced he was stepping down as party leader, touching off a leadership campaign.

With the opposition in some leadership turmoil, it is little wonder the Social Credit party sensed an opportunity to drive a new legislative highway through the BC political landscape. The first legislative session of the Thirty-third Parliament following the May 5 election began on June 23, 1983. The traditional pomp and ceremony gave no hint as to what the budget and its accompanying legislation might look like. When the government finally rolled out the budget and the twenty-six bills on July 7 and 8, Hanson remembers that the NDP caucus saw the package as the Social Credit's final assault on the achievements of Barrett's 1972–75 government. One former senior political Social Credit staffer says bluntly, "Everything was about the money and economic growth. No thought was given to social policy. The 1983 budget was a chance to get rid of the political opposition."

Whether the NDP announcement of its intention to filibuster the proposed legislation prompted the government to use twenty-four-hour legislative sittings, or whether the NDP announcement was a simply a reaction to the government's decision to hold round-the-clock sittings, can be debated at length. The fact is the government would do anything necessary to get its legislative package approved. According to recollections of former cabinet staff, Bennett and his cabinet colleagues "hated the GEU" and had decided on "open warfare" and an all-out assault to win their legislative and

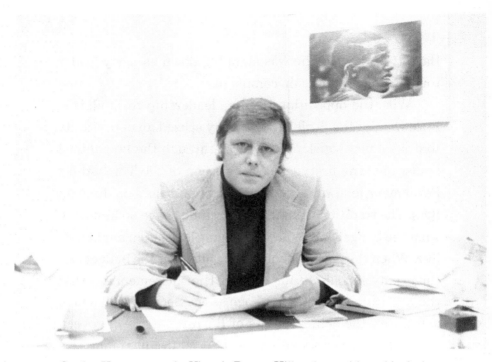

Gordon Hanson, MLA for Victoria-Beacon Hill and opposition whip during the 1983 Operation Solidarity legislative debates. BCGEU Archives

public relations battle. Both sides went into full battle mode and civility and common sense were immediate casualties.

Hanson outlines the NDP strategy by saying, "the NDP caucus realized our only strength was to hold the floor. It was decided to divide caucus into two teams each taking a twelve-hour shift in the House to participate in the round-the-clock legislative sessions." The two shifts were probably a wise course to pursue, as caucus members began to choose their party leadership preferences between popular non-caucus members David Vickers and Bill King. One shift in the legislature was led by Hanson, who was Bill King's campaign manager. The other shift was headed by MLA and former Barrett cabinet member Colin Gabelmann, who was David Vickers' campaign manager. Hanson described a "war on the floor" of the legislature. Both parties used every procedural trick in the book to advance their interests. The battle culminated in Barrett being ejected from the legislature, putting more pressure on the opposition caucus leadership team. He was physically dragged out of the legislative chamber by sergeant-at-arms staff and barred from returning for several months.

The opposition efforts were deeply appreciated by labour and community organizations. They needed an effective opposition to buy badly needed organizing time. Although the NDP leadership campaign proved to be a bit of a distraction, the caucus provided superb leadership opposing the government's agenda. The legislative battle as recorded in the July 1983 edition of Hansard is a priceless window on the public debate between the well-disciplined and professionally led Socreds intent on imposing a fiscally conservative agenda on BC versus class warfare–hardened social democrats intent on defending the social safety net for British Columbians. The parliamentary opposition slowed the government's progress significantly and allowed unions, citizens' organizations and community groups to organize a full-blown counterattack on the government. The labour plan was to use coordinated strike action as a central tactic. Since most of the largest bargaining units' collective agreements did not expire until the fall of 1983, other tactics requiring greater organizing efforts needed to be developed and implemented. From a labour point of view, the battle in the legislature and its accompanying media attention was an important aid to membership mobilization.

CHAPTER THREE

A UNION RESPONSE

G iven what was going on in Victoria, it was not surprising when the Ministry of Human Resources wanted to talk to the union about the future of Tranquille. It was required by the collective agreement. In the spring and summer of 1983, I was acting as the assistant director of collective bargaining and arbitration (CB and A) with the BCGEU. I had been hired on the servicing staff of the union in 1979, initially as a research officer and on assignment to do grievance arbitration for two components in the union. One of those components was the Social, Education and Health Services Component, known as Component 6, which had the bulk of its members employed by the Ministry of Human Resources (MHR). For this reason, I was well acquainted with the labour relations officials in the ministry.

The union's administrative structure was made up of three departments, each with a director and an assistant director. The CB and A department was the part of the union that dealt with contract administration matters and was expected to meet with government or its ministries on overall collective agreement administration and policy issues. My grievance-handling responsibilities with the Social, Education and Health Services Component made me a logical point of contact for MHR officials. Perhaps it was the laziness of summer or the government's legislative avalanche diverting my attention, but little did I suspect this meeting regarding Tranquille would be one I would never forget.

There are no notes as to what information the ministry staff relayed when they called my office to schedule a meeting but my diary for that day says only "Tranquille." The ministry proposed the meeting take place on July 19 at ministry offices. My office routinely agreed to the meeting. Although it was normal procedure for the MHR to contact me, the meeting was proposed on short notice and the ministry seemed to place great importance on it, at least by the cast of characters scheduled to attend on behalf of the ministry. Russell Dean was the director of human resources for the MHR. Terry Piper and Dick Butler were other senior managers in MHR. Butler was executive director of the Ministry and reported directly to deputy minister John Noble. To have all three of them at the meeting concerned me. I really wanted to have another union representative with me, preferably someone more familiar with Tranquille. But summer vacation meant there was no one else available on short notice to attend the meeting.

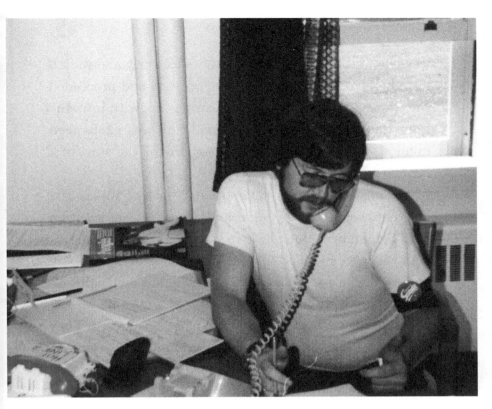

Gary Steeves at "BCGEU Headquarters" at Tranquille during the occupation. Gary Steeves

July 19, 1983 was a bright sunny summer Tuesday in Vancouver. The meeting was arranged for 2 p.m. in an MHR office on the west side of Vancouver, just off West Twelfth. The drive was a good half hour or so from my office at the best of times, but traffic could make it longer. I did not want to be late, so I left BCGEU's Burnaby headquarters early. Proceeding along the Grandview Highway to West Twelfth was pleasant. I arrived at the MHR office early and waited in the lobby. The meeting started on time and proceeded the way most labour relations meetings do, with introductions and handshakes. Some small talk was exchanged in an attempt to warm the atmosphere for the start of a serious meeting.

I joked that it was understandable why I was at the meeting because I was junior and would not get vacation until September. "But what are you guys, senior managers, doing at work in July?" I chided. The managers were stiff and uneasy in response. Something did not feel right. As the business part of the meeting started, the employer representatives outlined the need to close Tranquille. They explained that the ten-year plan announced by government in 1981 had been revised, scheduling the closure for December 31, 1984.

They reviewed the numbers, reminding me that there were 325 residents at Tranquille with 400 regular staff and 200 auxiliary employees (round figures they said). Then they pointed out that there were actually 475 regular established positions, but 75 were vacant. Management noted a declining need for residential spaces, deteriorating plant and equipment at the institution, and a growing ability to "return these patients" to their "community of origin." They said half the residents were from the Kamloops area, sixty were from the Okanagan, thirty-nine from Prince George and thirty were from the Kootenay area. These numbers are taken straight from my meeting notes of July 19, 1983, which reside in the BCGEU archives.

Management made an effort to appear sensitive to residents' needs. They said they would develop plans by the end of 1983, and that the Ministry of Lands, Parks and Housing would be providing 110 spaces in apartments and condos that could be subsidized for use by former residents of Tranquille. They said they would be looking to communities for proposals to house residents. I challenged or at least probed a little more deeply into each of the points being made by management. Some discussion followed but it was clear there were no plans for support services in the communities affected. Management confirmed that the budget currently before the legislature contained no provision for funding community resources and support services or societies that might house Tranquille residents. Management told me flatly that cost savings realized from the closure of Tranquille would be reallocated by government. It felt like a budget dump and a purely money-saving exercise.

It is fair to say that some of the discussion around operations and planning was necessitated by my limited knowledge of the specific details of Tranquille's operation. But the certainty in management's presentation indicated they had had extensive discussions before this meeting. I needed time to let these details sink in. As a union staff representative, I was trained to work within the rules established by the collective agreement. As the MHR officials droned on about their plans, or lack thereof, to close Tranquille, I accepted the government's right to cease operating a government program. The collective agreement recognized management's right to cease operating a public service—or to create a new one, for that matter. So my mind jumped to how the collective agreement might apply in these circumstances. When six hundred people employed at an institution are dismissed, what measures needed to be in place? Would the two hundred people classified as auxiliary employees face immediate layoff and severance pay? How many of the four hundred regular Tranquille employees would have more than three years' service in seniority and would therefore have to be offered alternate employment in the provincial public service? The size of the task in practical terms seemed daunting.

I asked about planning for redundant staff and management said they were "uncertain" about such arrangements. "No placement work has been done," but they were in "no hurry," they said. The meeting was becoming very negative in tone. I asked about the establishment of a joint committee pursuant to the provisions of the collective agreement. A joint committee, made up of management and union representatives, was a collective agreement mechanism to oversee layoff and recall procedures and deal with any issues that arose when a major reorganization or service discontinuation was happening. I asked about the application of

Treasury Board Order 57 that had been negotiated by the union for just these types of situations.

Management representatives immediately replied that they would like to work with Treasury Board Order 57 and the applicable provisions of the existing collective agreement between the government and the BCGEU. Articles of that collective agreement like 13.01 and 32.13 provided for a joint union–management committee to oversee the closure and transition of employees and reorganization mechanisms to assist the parties in a situation like a major program closure. But that was not the ministry's position, said Russell Dean. Management had received no direction from the minister or the deputy minister on this matter. Management essentially dismissed the notion of addressing employee issues. I immediately argued that the contract required a joint committee be set up and that Treasury Board Order 57 was legally binding.

Dean immediately pointed out that that would not be the case if Bill 2 and Bill 3, currently before the legislature, were passed into law. Bill 2 would amend the Public Service Labour Relations Act and eliminate the relevant collective agreement provisions that Tranquille employees would need to be fairly treated in an institutional closure. For example, it would render null and void most of the provisions of the collective agreement's layoff and recall rules. Layoff, recall, severance pay and no layoff protection would all be in the legal dust bin. A union recognition clause and a wage scale would be about all that was left of the collective agreement once the powers of Bill 2 were added to the provincial government arsenal.

Bill 3 would allow the government to terminate any public sector employee for any or no reason at all. What Dean was saying was that once the Social Credit's legislative attack on workers and their rights was completed, the closure of Tranquille would proceed and the employer would not owe employees so much as a handshake. I was shocked! I blurted out, "You mean you are going to fire six hundred workers in Kamloops?" The bosses looked nervously at each other and stared at me. No answer was required and nothing more needed to be said. I was completely stunned. Management's position was outrageous and disrespectful. I needed to call people with this astonishing news. What would the leadership of the union want to do? The ministry's position was madness and I needed to get back to union headquarters as soon as possible and see membership services director Jack Adams and collective bargaining and arbitration director Cliff Andstein.

I headed back to headquarters in my car. With no one to talk to, my mind was completely occupied with the what-ifs of the situation. How could a government suffering through a North American economic downturn think that terminating six hundred people was in anyone's best interest? The replay of the meeting rolled through my head like an old movie on an irritating loop. The warm summer sun was comforting but I was completely distracted. As I hurried along West Twelfth toward Burnaby, the traffic lights near Vancouver General Hospital turned from green to yellow as I continued through the intersection. A car turned left in front of me and the collision was unavoidable. I jumped out of the car and to my relief no one was injured. I quickly exchanged licence and phone numbers as well as home addresses with the other driver. The only injury was to my ability to get to the office as my front driver's side quarter panel was crushed into my front wheel. But the police officer attending bent over and pulled it back. I was on the road again and soon in Jack's office.

I explained to Jack and Cliff, in long, precise detail, the unbelievable plans of the ministry. They listened intently to the full story. Jack then said that I had better go to Kamloops and report to a full membership meeting that evening. The conversation immediately turned to strategy. After all, you could not drop a bombshell of information on the membership and then just leave town. "Oh, by the way you are all being fired and I have to catch a flight."

Jack Adams was a seasoned union leader and a Korean War veteran. He was quite strict and regimental in his demeanour. After his military service, he went to work in an east end Vancouver liquor store and became very active in the BC Government Employees' Association (BCGEA). He went on staff with the association/union and helped force the government into negotiating agreements before the

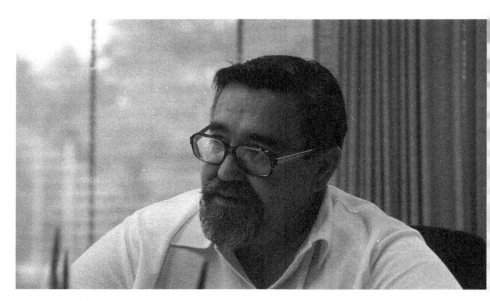

Jack Adams, director of the membership services department of the BCGEU.

union had legal bargaining rights. By 1983, he was one of the three departmental directors under General Secretary John Fryer. Jack was a powerful leader in both the union and the BC Federation of Labour. He was a brilliant tactician and strategist. As he thoughtfully stroked his goatee, he seemed to know exactly what buttons to press and what the government's reaction would be.

In the modern history of the union, the hiring of John Fryer as general secretary is generally regarded as the turning point to bona fide unionism in the provincial public service. Young pro-union leaders like Wayne Dermody, chair of the highways branch of the BCGEA and a member of the association's provincial executive (and later a staff representative with the BCGEU) fully supported the movement in the organization to leave the last vestiges of an association behind. The desire to change the association into a modern union resulted in a name change, a substantial increase in union staff, an expansion of the union's area-office network and a concerted campaign for full collective bargaining rights. Jack and Wayne were front and centre in these developments. Jack, as they say, knew where the bodies were buried. Jack Adams was a powerful leader: smart, blunt, direct and decisive. I listened intently to his advice, highly valuing his observations and opinions. When Jack suggested that the workers should stay after the general membership meeting and hold a sit-in protest, the concept of the occupation was born. It was up to me to deliver the news to the membership and organize the protest.

I had never been to Tranquille before. As my office made flight arrangements, I called the Kamloops area office staff representatives Dave McPherson and Al Lowndes. After the shock of calling a meeting on the employer's premises at II p.m. passed, we began discussing what needed to be done. It was agreed that building entrances may need to be secured if an occupation was to be effective. How to do so, however, was dependent on facts no one had. The type of doors, how they opened, how normal staff access could be maintained and many other considerations were among the unknowns. How members would react to the news was also unknown. Not knowing what members would want to do about it meant that we needed to prepare for any eventuality. I had read somewhere that breaking a straight section off a paper clip and sliding it into the door lock would prevent a key from being inserted into the door to unlock it. A small magnet could be used to remove the paper clip and the lock, undamaged, could be used as normal. As Al Lowndes loaded up on paper clips and small magnets, as well as rope, blank picket signs, felt markers and other materials we thought might be necessary that evening, I began thinking about what to say and how to say it. I gave up and decided to just tell members what transpired at the meeting blow by blow. Inspiration would just have to come on its own.

The airport in Kamloops is not far from Tranquille. Dave McPherson picked me up at the airport on his way to Tranquille and we discussed what might be expected at the meeting. McPherson described the efforts that had been made to reach local officers and shop stewards and the difficulty of reaching members on such short notice especially on a hot summer evening. Could a call to action fall flat due to lack of attendance?

The meeting was set for II p.m. It was an unusual meeting time and one that obviously piqued interest in the Tranquille BCGEU membership. Kamloops locals of the BCGEU were not considered the most militant locals in the union. The Kamloops membership was loyal, thoughtful and principled. They held strong opinions and were not afraid to express them. But they were not prone to act on the basis of wild rhetoric and they were certainly not mindlessly militant. They wanted the facts and thoughtful advice. As we approached Tranquille and entered the main dining hall, it was anyone's guess as to what the collective decision of the membership might be. The worst possible outcome might be a desire to wait and think about the situation. Dave McPherson was confident the workers would want action now. I was not so sure.

Dave McPherson was in his early thirties and one of the young staff representatives hired by Fryer as he expanded the union's organizing and servicing capability through a network of area offices around the province. Dave had been a brilliant student pursuing a science degree on a scholarship. He had taken a year off and gone to work in a Lower Mainland institution, got involved with the union and was hired by Fryer. He had a deep passion for social justice and loved organizing for social change. Politically active and engaged, he was involved with every aspect of the BCGEU local unions he worked with including those at Tranquille. His prediction of the emergency meeting's turnout was spot on as were most of his judgment calls.

Dave was a dream to work with. We clicked immediately and his creativity was such a bonus to every challenge we faced. No problem was too complicated and no solution unreachable for Dave. As we arrived, Dave seemed happy with the turnout. Hospital and Allied Services Local 205

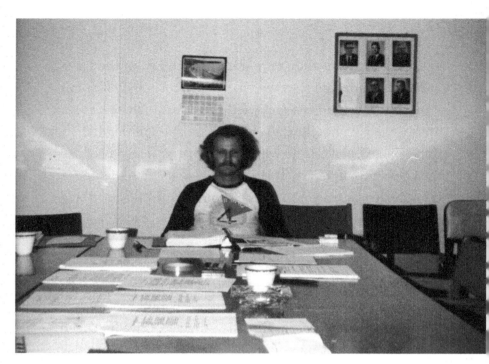

Dave McPherson at Tranquille during occupation. Gary Steeves

chairperson Bill Rhode was there as were most other local executive officers. A good portion of the steward body had turned out. Locals in the BCGEU were usually occupational groups with Local 205 (Hospital and Allied Services Component), the largest of the union locals at Tranquille. It was comprised of care aides, dietary staff, housekeeping staff and maintenance workers.

Bill Rhode called the meeting to order just after II p.m., a mere nine hours after my arrival at the MHR offices in Vancouver. He said the meeting was to hear about the government's plans for the future of Tranquille, as relayed to the union in a meeting that afternoon. The hall became very quiet as three hundred union members awaited my report. You could hear a pin drop as I rose to speak at the front of the dining hall.

I thanked Bill and apologized for meeting on such short notice. More pins dropped. I went step by step through the content of the meeting with ministry officials that afternoon. I tried to be as blunt and factual as I could. A few members in the front of the hall asked questions as I proceeded. Dave and I answered all the members' questions and I completed my report by saying, "The fact is that after October 31, they will likely be able to legally fire six hundred people." I then asked the members a question: "What is your choice? Do you want to accept the government's proposed disposition of Tranquille or do you want to fight back?" Toward the back of the hall a male member stood up and said in a loud clear voice, "We have no choice. What do you want us to do?" The membership stood and burst into an ovation that ended only after we asked everyone to sit back down.

The meeting instantly turned into an organizing and planning session. I explained that we thought occupying the buildings and refusing admittance to all non-union members including management was a good start. Dave took over. Buildings were designated for occupation, members scurried home to retrieve sleeping bags and pillows, sentries were designated and *Under New Management* signs were made. Each building and/or department of the institution established their own occupation schedules. Sentries were needed at all doorways and sleeping spaces were identified and occupied. Workers in each work unit spent sixteen hours a day at work—eight working and eight sleeping—and sentries maintained twenty-four-hour coverage of occupied areas. The closure of Tranquille had been proposed and the union in its most democratic form had reacted. There would be no easy way out for anyone.

CHAPTER FOUR

FROM DOMINANCE
TO DEMISE

The cabinet of BC was well along in its plans to dramatically and permanently abandon the use of large institutions for the care of people with developmental challenges. The use of institutions like Woodlands, Glendale and Tranquille was a major and important element in carrying out government policy pertaining to the care of persons who were developmentally delayed. Riverview Hospital played a similar role in the policy and care of people with mental health challenges. To contemplate the closure of Tranquille was a huge step on the path to deinstitutionalization of care and a departure from nearly one hundred years of public policy direction on the care of the persons with some type of mental disability.

When Tranquille opened in 1906 as a tuberculosis (TB) sanatorium, the BC Anti-Tuberculosis Society was searching for land somewhere in the province's dry belt as the ravages of TB took its toll in BC. They approached the Fortune family

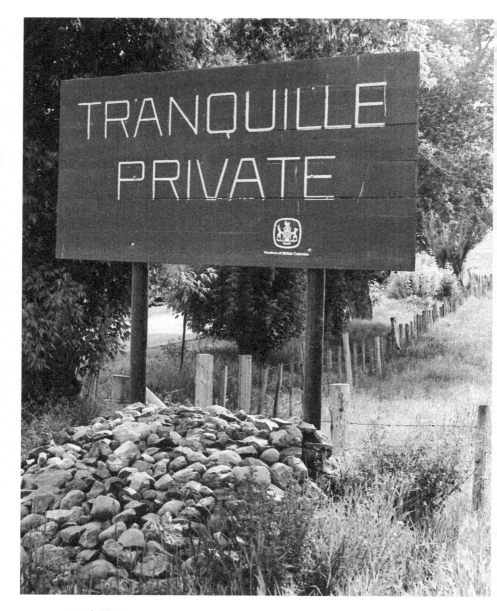

BCGEU Archives

who owned an expansive ranch on the Tranquille River just outside Kamloops. The land was purchased and the Kamloops Board of Trade supported the construction of a sanatorium. It was opened in 1907 and operated privately as the King Edward Sanatorium.

Tuberculosis has been present in humans since antiquity. It was a major cause of death and the most prevalent human affliction for centuries. In the first couple of decades of the nineteenth century, TB continued to be the virulent killer it had been. In 1800, 25 percent of all deaths in Europe were due to tuberculosis. In the United Kingdom, one in four deaths were due to what they called "consumption," the common term for tuberculosis at that time. The situation improved gradually after the major discovery, in 1820, that TB was a single disease.

Tuberculosis continued to be a major life-threatening disease well into the twentieth century. In 1918 France, for example, one in six deaths was caused by TB. In 1906, the year of Tranquille's construction, Albert Calmette and Camille Guérin achieved the first genuine success in immunization by using attenuated bovine-strain tuberculosis. But the prevalence of the disease had generated enormous public attention and people demanded unprecedented government action. In British Columbia, part of the government's response was to convert private-care facilities or sanatoriums into public healthcare facilities. In the political parlance of the 1960s and '70s, the government's action could be described as nationalizing private enterprise. Tranquille had operated as a private sanatorium for one and a half decades before the provincial government purchased the property in 1921. The government immediately assumed operation of Tranquille upon purchase of the private sanatorium, and the following year acquired the neighbouring Cooney Ranch. The newly purchased ranch was amalgamated with the Tranquille property and expanded the sanatorium's operation. Almost overnight, Tranquille became a major source of economic and financial benefit to the Kamloops area, due in large measure to the extensive farm operations carried out on sanatorium property.

The government was no stranger to running institutions. After British Columbia ceased the practice of deporting "male lunatics" to the Napa Asylum in California in the 1860s and joined Canada in 1871, its institutions formed a significant part of British Columbia's healthcare system especially as it pertained to people with mental health issues or people who were developmentally delayed. It opened the Victoria Asylum for the Insane in 1872 and the Provincial Lunatic Asylum in 1878 in New Westminster. The government later renamed the New West institution the Public Hospital for the Insane. It served people with intellectual and developmental disabilities, and in 1950 was renamed Woodlands School. In 1920, the Public Hospital for the Insane was given a mandate of custodial care for the "feeble minded." It advanced a mandate to educate children with intellectual disabilities. Woodlands School closed in 1996.

For more than one hundred years, the government of British Columbia used institutions as a foundational tool in their public health policy toolkit. The distinction between people with mental health challenges and people with intellectual challenges was not clearly defined by governments of the early twentieth century. BC's provincial government, however, did make distinctions in their institutions between people requiring medical attention and people who were developmentally delayed. The latter required special education and life-skills training, which the government had provided through residential schools. The government demonstrated its understanding of mental health and its reliance on institutions by opening the Hospital for the Mind in Coquitlam in 1913. It later became known as Essondale, and eventually Riverview Hospital.

The government's reliance on institutions as an important tool for the delivery of social and health policy reached its zenith with the opening of Glendale Lodge near Victoria in 1976. It provided a residential care facility for people on Vancouver Island who were developmentally delayed. It was the last of the government's large institutions to house and educate persons with developmental disabilities. Its opening also demonstrated how long the government clung to its institutional policy direction for care of people with developmental disabilities and those suffering from a mental illness.

By the late 1970s, the BC government operated many facilities addressing a variety of health conditions and situations. Some were in large centres, such as Pearson Hospital in Vancouver, where their social and economic impact was not as obvious as institutions in smaller communities, such as Dellview in Vernon and Skeenaview Lodge in Terrace.

The BC government's policy direction of caring for people with developmental disabilities and those with some type of mental illness by using residential institutions was mainly driven by the lack of an alternative. The absence of any other health or social service care system in the province to address the needs of institutional residents and their families was a fact of life. Acute-care hospitals and emergency rooms were completely incapable of handling people with mental health issues. The medical care model was unsuited for people with intellectual challenges, and the primary caregivers were the families of both the mentally ill and the developmentally disabled. The BC government's use of institutions was partly aimed at relieving the care burden on these families. In reality, relief for caregivers unable to cope with the multitude of care issues in their families was an important aspect of the government's response to the needs of the developmentally disabled. There were other practical factors that came to shape government policy directions, but institutionalization continued as an extensive and expensive centrepiece of provincial health and social services care policies until government restraint hit the cabinet table in the early 1980s.

Government spending restraint was a political issue that would severely impact Tranquille. The Tranquille story of service, however, had encountered previous bumps in the road. In the mid 1950s, the tuberculosis crisis had subsided. The post-war development of new antibiotics, improved immunization and more effective treatment combined to reduce the patient population at the Tranquille Sanatorium. The decline in population prompted the provincial government to announce the closure of the sanatorium in 1958. The proposal to close Tranquille hit the Kamloops area hard and created a huge outcry. The business community in particular was very upset. After all, the new W.A.C. Bennett Social Credit government was supposed to be a friend of business. Tranquille was a very significant economic, political and social influence on the city and was an important employment engine for the Thompson-Nicola region. The thought of Tranquille's closure alarmed key local decision-makers, particularly as potential losses of income were calculated and individual business impacts were identified. Tranquille was the third largest employer in the city and was intricately linked to the regional economy—a fact that would remain a part of life for nearly three more decades.

The political uproar about the proposed Tranquille closure brought the merchants and citizens of Kamloops into sharp conflict with W.A.C. Bennett's local MLA and

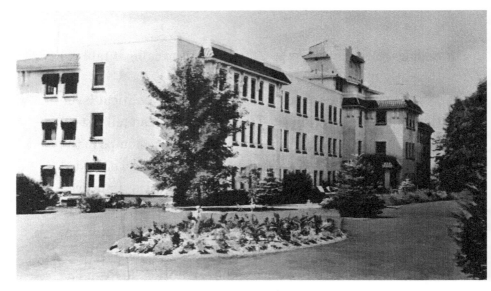

Historical photo of the Greaves Building at Tranquille. BCGEU Archives

Social Credit cabinet minister Phil Gaglardi. Gaglardi was in real political trouble and searched desperately for a solution. Such angst was generated politically in Kamloops that no solution was off the table. Woodlands School in New Westminster was overcrowded, so Gaglardi convinced the provincial cabinet that Tranquille could relieve the pressure.

The W.A.C. Bennett government announced the transfer of the Tranquille Sanatorium to the provincial Mental Health Services Branch. It was retained and refurbished as a facility for people Premier Bennett referred to as "mentally retarded." Note that the use of language to stigmatize developmentally delayed people changed little from the stark language of the early twentieth century until the early

1980s. In fact, in 1983, advocates and family of Tranquille residents still called their organization the Kamloops Society for the Mentally Handicapped. For W.A.C. Bennett in 1958, terminology was less important than saving his minister of transportation. Gaglardi's rationale of relieving the overcrowding at Woodlands School worked for Bennett and the Social Credit cabinet. Although the solution made sense given the overcrowded circumstances at Woodlands, everyone knew that Gaglardi's electoral survival was the real issue. Tranquille took on the mandate, as set out by the Mental Health Services Branch, to provide life-skills training to the residents of Tranquille. Mildly and moderately developmentally delayed individuals were moved into the beautiful rural setting of Tranquille and an education model was fully implemented.

According to Diane Purvey, author of *Thrown Out into the Community: The Closure of Tranquille*, the institution in 1958 was made up of over forty buildings, four of which were designated as hospitals. There were cottages for doctors' housing, a fire hall, a kitchen, an industrial laundry, farm buildings, nurses' buildings and residential dormitories. A power plant supplied the institution's power needs and a system of underground tunnels connected the main buildings. Over the years, Tranquille had a peak resident population of seven hundred with a mandate to serve the interior and north of British Columbia. The care of residents focused, in a residential setting, on training and habilitating people with the potential to live in the community. This focus resulted in another change that care staff could neither foresee nor predict.

From 1971 to 1983, four hundred residents were deinstitutionalized from Tranquille and placed in community settings. Tranquille's track record proved that the training model of care was very effective. The departing residents were mainly replaced by new residents from other provincial institutions, including Woodlands. The incoming residents were more severely or profoundly disabled, requiring more extensive, personal and permanent care. Tranquille's success in the 1970s resulted in a resident population quite different from the Tranquille population of the 1950s and 1960s. In 1983, Tranquille director of nursing Alex McIntosh classified 80 percent of residents in his institution as "profoundly retarded," in need of "segregated, protective, custodial environments." Tranquille was now caring for people whose transition to the community was a much more difficult process than previous placements. The training model was losing some of its relevance and any plan to close the institution became much more challenging.

As the issue of government restraint generated cabinet table discussions in the early eighties, serious thought was given to how it might be achieved. In 1982, the provincial treasury board presented cabinet with a document outlining public service staff reductions for 1983. The cabinet had decided to reduce the civil service by 25 percent across the board and the presentation to cabinet said, "a major reduction in the staff in the institutions at this time would jeopardize the overall plan toward decentralized care of the mentally retarded. Therefore, the ministry is proposing only a 12 percent staff cutback at this time with institutions effectively being exempt from the current manpower objectives until the planning with respect to decentralization and community resources is completed." It summarized that "because the majority of services provided by the ministry of human resources are mandated under legislation related to income security and family and children services, it is not possible to meet the 75 percent staffing targets."

It is worthy of note that the treasury board document did not use the term "deinstitutionalization." The document instead referred to the government's plan for ministry of human resources institutions as "decentralization" and recognized the possible need for community resources to support decentralization. The notion of an improved quality of life for residents of MHR institutions was not specified as the public policy goal. The structure of the care system was the real issue for cabinet. This was, judging by the rest of the treasury board document, based on the cabinet's determination to reduce staffing costs and achieve budget goals.

The secret discussions leading to the decision by cabinet to close Tranquille signalled more than a shift in its hundred-year-old mental healthcare model. The preparations did not consider the history or current realities of

Tranquille, its economic role in the region nor its role in supporting mentally fragile people. A careful review of cabinet documents between 1982 and 1986 suggests that nothing but staffing and budget considerations were evaluated by cabinet committees and the full body of cabinet itself as decisions on the future of Tranquille were made. Beginning with civil services staffing reductions in 1982, the Ministry of Human Resources as previously mentioned had difficulty meeting the arbitrary reduction figures. Statutory obligations to families and children meant other measures were required to meet the arbitrary staffing-reduction target of 25 percent. The services provided by people in ministry-run institutions like Tranquille also made staffing cuts difficult, but the closure of a major institution would be a big and necessary leap toward reducing the size of government and the size of the ministry's budget.

Cabinet meeting records routinely show reports on how various ministries were doing with reaching their reduction targets. One such report in January 1983 alerted cabinet to problems with reducing the size of the public service: "if the government desires certainty respecting its rights to reduce the public service in accordance with these plans, legislation will be required." It is the first indication, in writing, of the massive legislative assault that would come six months later. The same memo noted, "There are only two ministries where there is a medium or high risk that their staff reductions cannot be achieved because of restrictions in the collective agreement." It named the ministries of human resources and the attorney general.

A footnote entitled "Regarding Tranquille" said, "The risk can be considered medium because there are good arguments that the major reason for the change is based on social policy considerations. The high-risk aspects reflect the numbers of employees involved." The Tranquille employee population was cited earlier in the report as five hundred. The

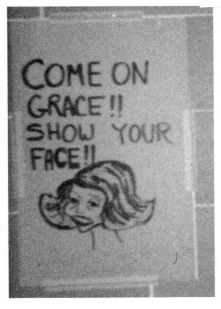

Signs included political messages to Minister Grace McCarthy.

Gary Steeves

cabinet was aware that a decision to close the Tranquille institution would help achieve civil service reduction goals but would also be in keeping with social trends of the time. Between 1965 and 1980, fifty thousand psychiatric hospital beds in Canadian facilities were closed following a general worldwide trend away from institutional care and toward community-based care models. These trends were based on civil libertarian beliefs and humanistic reforms, a newly reinforced belief in social integration and improved medications in the treatment of mental health issues.

BC's Social Credit government wanted to run a spring 1983 election on government restraint. Reducing the number of provincial government employees by 25 percent was a critical piece of their campaign vision. The cabinet's neoliberal conservatism and the lack of a real understanding of the needs of people with disabilities were dominant conditions in the Social Credit analysis of vulnerable British Columbians. The nearly hundred-year dominance of institutions in provincial health and social-service policy was justifiably in decline. The demise of important care resources for vulnerable individuals, however, was not a concern for Social Credit bean-counters and ideologues. And other financial preparations were being made to position the 1983 provincial election restraint campaign for Bennett and his Socreds.

Cabinet had forged ahead, accepting the political support of social reformers. The November 27, 1981 press release by the British Columbia Association for the Mentally Retarded praised Premier Bill Bennett as he "announced the phase-out of institutions for the mentally retarded, and a commitment by the government to the principle of community living for mentally handicapped persons." Elise Clark, president, went on to say, "The Throne Speech announcement of a coordinated government approach to programs and services means that all mentally handicapped persons will be able to enjoy a way of life most of us take for granted: the ability to live in your own community, with access to housing, health, education, and recreation facilities and programs."

The government had not the least intention of putting the enormous savings from institutional cuts back into a community care system. In fact, subsequent cabinet documents show the deliberate decision taken by cabinet to prohibit reinvestment of savings in a government-supported community care system. The cabinet forced ministries to put "savings from employee expenditures" back into general revenue. A cabinet report noted, "Tranquille—approximately five hundred employees involved—targeted for completion by December 31, 1984. Proposal is to transfer the residents to non-profit societies and facilities run by independent contractors."

The government set financial and staffing goals before any assessment of the needs of Tranquille residents was done. The only plans government made for Tranquille employees was to eliminate any benefits they may have had under their collective agreement and Treasury Board Order 57. The evolution of the Social Credit Party and the fruition of its old-fashioned conservatism would lead British Columbians to the brink of chaos. Money has a way of driving people to odd places. In this case, cabinet ministers were simply blind to the needs of people with intellectual challenges and their professional caregivers. The cabinet was reminded often of the need for legislation to get past legal and contractual obligations to their employees.

Skeenaview Lodge was an example they referred to regularly. The 126 employees remained on the payroll for an extended period after the institution had closed. According to a treasury board report, a majority of them would likely be placed in the society-run facility scheduled to open in February 1984 while others would have to be moved. Staffing plans of the treasury board took the collective agreement obligations to employees into account but the cabinet saw the collective agreement with the BCGEU as an impediment to quick and easy downsizing. But Bills 2 and 3 could save the government from being responsible in any way to displaced workers. And Tranquille workers could be among the first of those negatively impacted.

Residents, too, would be among those damaged by the legislation. Staffing cuts would lead to a disruption of the continuity of care by disrupting the care team/resident relationship. The dominance of provincial institutions for the delivery of health and social service programs was on a path to complete demise. That path was being engineered and constructed by BC's Social Credit Party and their philosophical belief that market conditions and community benevolence were the important hallmarks of society. Governments, by contrast, were responsible for keeping government small and pushing services onto communities who would provide those thought to be necessary. A closer look at Social Credit and their anti-social, pro-business attitude explains much about how Tranquille—its employees, its residents and their families—were treated in 1983.

The Social Credit's decision to move away from the use of residential institutions in caring for persons with developmental disabilities was a huge shift in public policy. Social Credit was motivated by cost considerations and the size of its payroll. Social Credit felt its only obligation was to keep private enterprise afloat during the devastating international recession and the only way to do so was by acting as a reliable source of financial support for BC industry. If governments could aid the money-making companies to provide jobs around the province, then BC might emerge from the recession in a strong financial position. But that meant restricting government spending on government bureaucracy and channelling funds to private enterprise. Cabinet records of decisions for 1982 until 1988 are full of decisions to give grants, loans and tax relief to private corporations while aid to the poor and disabled was reviewed, capped or ignored. The Social Credit vision was, as Kurt Vonnegut told the graduating class of Bennington College in 1970, "just too hard on the old, the sick and those that do not have that certain something that Nelson Rockefeller has in such abundance." Advocates for the developmentally disabled would learn that lesson a few years down the road. As the legislative battle raged on, union members at Tranquille began running a large and complex institution without the participation of management. The opposition to Bill Bennett and his government had opened another front in the struggle for fair treatment.

CHAPTER FIVE

RUNNING THE INSTITUTION

When the government overplayed its hand on the closure of Tranquille, months ahead of the passage of the legislation and the expiry of the collective agreements, the BCGEU was handed a huge opportunity to fight the government's agenda. Shock and awareness spread rapidly among union members and the public. The budget and the accompanying twenty-six pieces of legislation were studied in exacting detail and the longer the look, the more shock and alarm was generated in unions and liberal academia.

The sudden late-night union meeting at Tranquille on Tuesday, June 19 had ignited a wave of action and a sleepless night for Dave McPherson and me. The social work conference room had been designated as my sleeping place. It had a small office in one corner of the room with a phone. At about eight o'clock in the morning of the twentieth, Dave and I phoned Jack Adams at his office at BCGEU headquarters to bring him up to date on the overnight developments.

Following the conversation, Dave and I proceeded to the dining hall for much-needed coffee.

An assessment of what had been decided and what needed to be done was required. Planning ahead seemed out of the question, as just keeping up with what the membership was doing and coordinating the fledgling takeover seemed more than enough to think about. As I am reported to have said in *The Province*, the occupation "could last all day at least." By July 20, the media, too, had caught up to the story. Reporters were at the institution in numbers and a horde followed Dave and me almost everywhere we went. The news crews were from every national outlet. There were TV news crews from CBC, BCTV and CTV. There were local Kamloops radio and newspaper reporters, as well as newspaper reporters from the Lower Mainland. It was quite a mob in the beginning and every move around the institution was a scrum.

In our phone conversation with Jack, Dave and I were struck by his questions as to whether or not we had talked to the RCMP. We told Jack that we had not. We told Jack we had not even seen any police around let alone talked to them. He said that apparently there was an intense back-and-forth going on between the premier's office and RCMP. According to Robbie Robinson, BCGEU communications officer at the time and the union's contact to deal with the RCMP, the premier's office wanted the union trespassers arrested. Robbie had apparently already been contacted by the RCMP in their attempts to find out what was going on and was consequently involved in lengthy discussions with the RCMP's union liaison officer. In subsequent discussions, Robbie advanced the argument that no harm was being done and no laws were being broken. He further argued that it was all political and the RCMP might not want to get caught in the middle of a political dispute.

Stay tuned, Jack had told us. We worried for a split second and then realized we had so much to do that getting arrested might not be the worst thing that could happen. BCGEU headquarters wanted reports. The media wanted every ounce of news that could be generated. The Ministry of Human Resources wanted to meet secretly away from the institution and the premier wanted us arrested. Dave and I were more concerned with the state of the occupation but we needed to keep reporters engaged and telling our story. The tasks ahead did not look simple.

The initial step in the occupation was to take over the administration offices, which meant two buildings where about twenty-five union members worked. Management and any non-union members were barred entry. Sentries were at the doors and the administrative/clerical staff worked a shift and slept a shift so the office had twenty-four-hour coverage. Local union activists had set up a scheduling bureau to figure out who was on duty when and who was doing what; and ensured that new signage was in place at the two administrative buildings. The *Under New Management* signs served as the workers' declaration that they strongly disagreed with the provincial government and supported the union's actions.

Notwithstanding my comments in *The Province*, the workers were not changing their minds. It seemed that members remained committed to what they had decided the night before. Wherever I went the morning of the twentieth, I was met with supportive comments and suggestions for continued militancy. Often the intensity of a meeting is gone by the next morning but that was not the case at Tranquille. Many of the rank-and-file members wanted the bosses expelled and more operational areas occupied. The cafeteria, canteen, laundry and power plants, as well as the fire department and the farm operations, were all yet to be taken and the media kept asking, "What will you do next?"

Over coffee in the dining hall on July 20, Dave McPherson and I reviewed, with satisfaction, what had been done. We turned our attention to the future. If we were to continue the occupation beyond the two administrative buildings and the twenty-five or so affected union members, there were a number of things we needed to do. We needed to expand the number of buildings and institutional space controlled by the union. We needed to demonstrate and reinforce the notion that residents were not in any peril from the union's occupation. We needed to educate the public on what the Province of BC should do for the residents of Tranquille if a transition to the community was in fact to be carried out

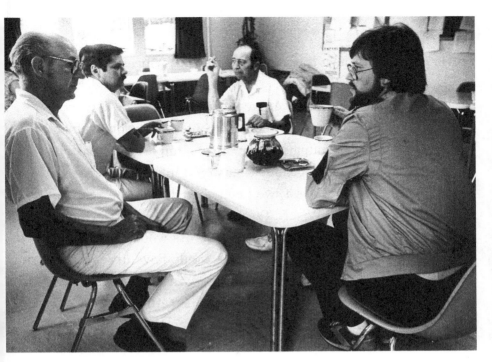

Gary Steeves in the kitchen talking to dietary workers during the occupation. BCGEU Archives

successfully, and we had to set up an internal governance structure to run the occupation.

That was pretty much our agenda as we finished our coffee. It seemed straightforward. We convened a meeting of local executive members in the administration board-room. It was one of the occupied buildings and housed the psychology and social work departments. We turned it into the BCGEU headquarters during the occupation and it was, incidentally, the room where I slept on the floor. We would continue to meet there each evening at 7 p.m. as the occupation continued.

On July 20, however, we met at noon. As the local executives and union staff filled the conference room to meet as an ad hoc occupation committee, important decisions had to be made, decisions that would inform our work for the days ahead. First, we needed to decide the scope of the occupation. Wisely, the leadership group determined that the living wards of the residents would not be subject to occupation. Management would have unrestricted access to the so-called healthcare wards. This was a wise decision because it helped us demonstrate the safety and good care residents continued to receive during the occupation. It cannot be overemphasized how concerned we were about the quality of care and how devastating to our cause it would be if something drastic were to happen to a resident. As the occupation continued, we arranged a number of things designed to demonstrate the workers' competence as caregivers. Tours of the institution by journalists and visits by our member of parliament were two of these activities. Next, the ad hoc committee decided to expand the occupation each day until all non-care buildings were "under new management." These first two decisions were unanimous and required remarkably little debate or discussion.

Education of the public as to the needs of Tranquille residents was high on the agenda. It was inextricably linked to the first concern about quality care during the occupa-tion. Almost every worker at Tranquille felt that the care of residents was at least as important as what would happen to themselves as employees. At times, it was a challenge to get workers to concentrate on their own issues because all they wanted to discuss was what would happen to our residents. One healthcare worker said to me that getting an evalua-tion and placement plan developed for residents was all the workers needed to focus on because it was the union's job to look after employees. I said that was fine but the employees were the union and the leadership had to advocate for both residents and employees.

I was struck by the exchange because this healthcare worker so deeply trusted the union to look after her. She made it very clear that nothing was going to stop her from fighting the ministry over how helpless residents were about to be treated. To her, placement in the community was one step from living on the street and she was not going let her residents be put into jeopardy without a fight. I was so impressed with her attitude and proud to work for a union with members like her. I was even more gratified to find her view was fairly typical of union members at Tranquille. What a group they were! Public education as to the plight of Tranquille residents had to be done through the media and there were lots of them around. An education plan was needed and a committee of union members went to work on the issue.

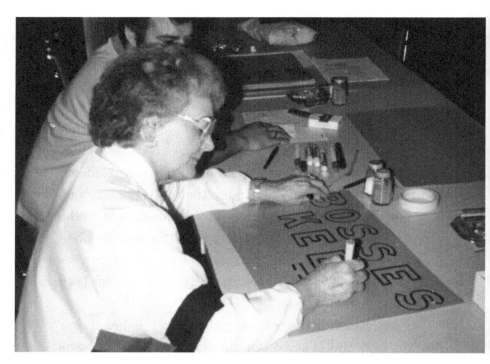

Union members making occupation signs. Gary Steeves

While the meeting was proceeding in the administrative boardroom, Dave McPherson was strangely absent from the big table. At one point when his input was needed in order to facilitate an important discussion, I impatiently snapped, "Where is Dave?"

"Over here," he said from the floor in the corner of the room. I could not believe my eyes! He was on his hands and knees and he had a pale blue bedsheet, a Styrofoam coffee cup and a black felt marker in hand. He was just finishing production of a BCGEU flag. The large dogwood logo, perfectly shaped, was in the centre of the sheet and was amazingly good. He stood up holding the flag. "We should put this up in place of the province's flag at the fire hall," he said. Everyone began talking at once. Excitement broke out. So much for the meeting. We all trooped outside and as we walked across the yard from the East Pavilion to the fire hall, the media contingent fell in behind. They recorded members gathering around as we lowered the provincial flag and raised the BCGEU flag to loud cheers. I made a brief speech about defying the government and sending a message to Premier Bennett, or something to that effect. It was the most exciting thing we could have done in an otherwise action-packed day.

On July 20, I was worried about bringing control and order to our actions but Dave McPherson was about generating excitement and media coverage. Thank goodness for the Dave McPhersons of the world. I learned a number of lessons from Tranquille, and Dave taught me most of them. The day was not over yet, however, and the decisions on governance needed membership affirmation. A general membership meeting was scheduled for 7 p.m. and the fundamental question as to whether or not to continue the occupation was on the agenda. No sense setting up a governance structure, an education program, or demonstrating how well we were meeting the needs of residents if the occupation was to end. As meeting time approached, more than three hundred members, over half of all the BCGEU employed at Tranquille, crowded into the dining hall. The day was to get even busier.

Bill Rhode, chair of BCGEU local 205, the largest BCGEU local in the Kamloops area, called the meeting to order. Bill was a good chairperson. He was calm, stoic and alert, and not much got past him. It became clear very quickly that members had no intention of stopping the occupation. The meeting atmosphere matched the reaction of the world around the institution. Kamloops was thrilled that someone was standing up for the area's interests. If you worked at Tranquille, people on the street held you in some esteem as being a cross between a revolutionary hero and a strategic genius. People would stop you on the street and ask with excitement in their voice and amazement on their face, "What's going on out there?" When the reply was, "A protest against this government," a "Right on!" was usually the response.

As I recall, the July 20 meeting was fairly self-congratulatory. Bill Rhode was low-key and businesslike and the membership thanked the leadership for the decisions and recommendations the ad hoc committee had made earlier in the day and brought forward to this evening's meeting. I do not recall a dissenting voice on the question of whether or not to continue the occupation. Deputy Minister Noble's letter to BCGEU President Norm Richards was at the centre of discussions as most members wanted to know what would happen to the residents. The letter was clearly slim on details about any planning processes for either residents or employees. Grace McCarthy's newsworthy comments that day in Victoria that her ministry would "try to relocate as many as possible" provided little comfort to residents, their advocates or their caregivers.

To put an exclamation mark on the determination to continue the occupation, members endorsed occupying the kitchen and dining facilities. Designating these areas added them to the restricted, union-only list of buildings on the institution's grounds. These facilities were placed "under new management," which added sixty-five union members to the occupation roster. Members were very pleased about the recommendation to leave residents' sleeping dorms alone and continue to allow management to visit the residents' living wards. But the expansion of geographic space meant managers had fewer areas to enter and no access to food and drink from the kitchens they no longer supervised. Management soon retreated to a small office in the village and were later moved to a small cottage, with no furniture and no air conditioning, located at the western edge of the property. Sitting on the floor in their business attire—dress suits in the case of men—made a curious sight each day as I brought over the documents the union members required them to sign.

At the 7 p.m. general membership meeting, we also reported the results of our meeting with Tranquille manager Terry Prysiazniuk earlier that day. When I took a pile of documents to sign to the managers in their cottage, the general manager and I sat at a picnic table for a chat. Some management staff and a couple of union representatives were there as well. The issues the union was pursuing, and my five questions, were outside of his sphere of responsibility, Prysiazniuk said. I soon recognized that it was unfair to press him on those issues. When the ministry would start assessments of resident needs for community placement, and how redundancy placements and job offers for employees would take place, were outside of his knowledge and control. Such matters were controlled by MHR headquarters because the issues were really to do with ministry budgets, not the care of residents. We agreed to meet the next day after we consulted with our respective senior officials.

In my view, the most important decision of the general membership meeting was the decision to approve the establishment of an ad hoc committee to guide the membership in the establishment of a "new management committee" to run the institution. The ad hoc group of local union leaders got to work immediately and would make recommendations within a few days. That a governance structure was to be established was very good news for me. Since my meeting only the day before in Vancouver, Dave and I had been the primary decision-makers after consulting with local union executives. And even though local executives, steward bodies and the general membership had been fully participating, an elected committee was needed to deal with occupation issues going forward. There simply is no substitute for a

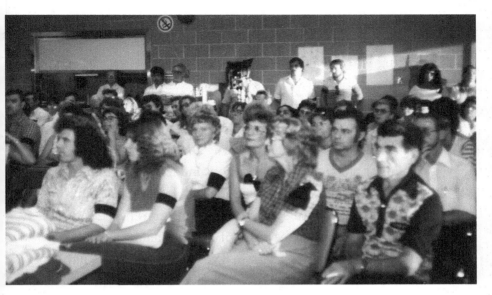

General meeting of members at Tranquille, July 1983. There was one almost every night during the occupation. Gary Steeves

representative democracy. The Greek city-state model of decision-making with general membership meetings every night had a limited shelf life.

July 20 was the first full day of the occupation and quite a day it was. The occupation had been solidified and structured to make sure it could expand without impacting resident care. A governing body to facilitate union members running the institution was being worked out. A new flag flew over the institution, and public education initiatives were being developed. Most importantly, the union members at Tranquille were doing all of this through a democratic structure using democratic methods and principles. A meeting with local management representatives had even been worked into the day's busy schedule so there was no misunderstanding on their part as to the intentions of the union and its membership groups. As the occupation progressed, it became evident that the government just did not care about getting the institution under management control. Were the union members doing too good a job of running the institution, or was government just unprepared for the necessary steps to close the institution? What unfolded next did not cast the government in a very compassionate light.

CHAPTER SIX

LEGAL THREATS

W ithin a couple of days of the occupation, the protest had taken on a life of its own. By July 24, with the occupation in full swing, progress was being made on all of the key issues the ad hoc group of leaders had set out to address. BCGEU members and their elected leaders had made a number of important decisions to set a foundation for future decision-making bodies to lead the occupation. The establishment of a governance structure could not happen soon enough, in my opinion. A number of working groups or committees were established to deal with everything from an in-house newspaper called the *Tranquille Tough Times* to public education around services needed by persons with developmental disabilities. Media scrutiny of the union's occupation activities was intense.

As the occupation matured in the days ahead, the best single method of getting a story out was to call Kamloops newsman Angelo Iacobucci. He was incredible. He was always available and would put stories out on his radio network in machine-like fashion. I really liked Angelo and was deeply saddened by his passing in 2018. I do not remember all the media folks by name and face but the list I had in my binder during the occupation was long and contained many household names with home phone numbers. No one, it seemed, wanted to miss a development in the quickly evolving story. The BCGEU received extensive media coverage, and the whole fiasco was blamed on the Social Credit government. Both public events and behind-the-scenes activity were investigated and usually covered in detail.

Although the number of news crews declined over the week, the reporters' desire to monitor and report on any new development had not subsided. Understandably, the reporting became more businesslike and less frenzied than the coverage had been at the beginning of the occupation. The media showed more interest in background stories even though the scope of the occupation had expanded daily. A major portion of the news coverage centred on the duelling letters between BCGEU president Norm Richards and MHR deputy minister John Noble.

On July 20, the deputy minister had quickly written to President Richards saying he wished to confirm information provided "to your representative in a ministry-initiated meeting" on July 19, 1983. "The Ministry of Human Resources will be establishing a planned process for the closing of Tranquille including consultation with the unions and with

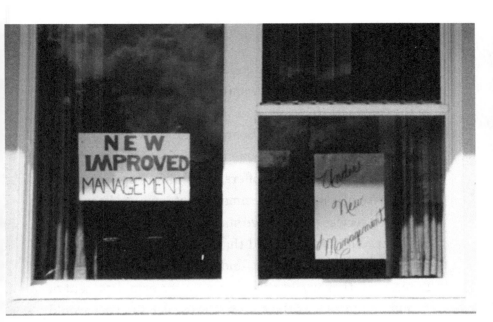

Signs indicating that Tranquille was "under new management" during the occupation. Gary Steeves

due regard for provisions of the collective agreements." I must admit that it felt a bit like the ministry trying to say, "Steeves got it wrong." I know I got it right and a review of my meeting notes thirty-five years later confirm even the worst interpretation. Noble was engaging in gamesmanship that to me was despicable. For a government ministry charged with the care of extremely vulnerable British Columbians, engaging in such behaviour was beyond my comprehension.

Noble's boss, Grace McCarthy, also said publicly and repeatedly, "We will consult once the occupation ends." The union, of course, did not see consultation as the starting point. For the BCGEU, our collective agreements were the starting points. The union wanted the terms and conditions of the contracts to be followed, including any applicable side agreements like Treasury Board Order 57, which provided for a number of practical benefits such as early retirement credits, public service job offers and training opportunities in the case of a major government shutdown or discontinuation of a service where large staff reductions were involved.

Our analysis concluded that if the ministry was going to consult with the union under the existing collective agreement, they would have agreed to the establishment of a joint committee as the contract provided and they would have routinely agreed to the application of Treasury Board Order 57 at our July 19 meeting. The fact that management failed to do so suggested they had other plans in mind. Russell Dean's statement in our July 19 meeting about delaying staff planning until after the outcome of Bills 2 and 3 was determined by the legislature said it all. The ministry knew that Bill 2 would wipe out virtually all collective agreement benefits and protections for Tranquille workers while Bill 3 would give government the right to fire any worker for any reason.

President Richards replied to Noble's July 20 letter the same day saying, "the union was advised that the ministry could give no commitment regarding continued compliance with the Master and Component Agreements since there was an 'air of uncertainty due to the pending legislation.'"

Richards' very detailed letter stated the union had "asked if that meant the ministry would sit and wait until legislation, which nullifies our collective agreement, is passed." The union was obviously alarmed as it noted the ministry's reply. Ministry officials said they "had no mandate to discuss that issue." Richards' demand in the letter was blunt. He said that the union wanted "a written commit-

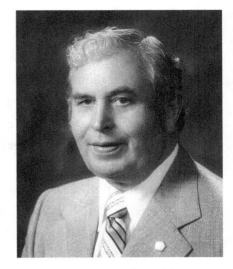

Norm Richards, president of the BCGEU. BCGEU Archives

ment from the minister that the provisions of the collective agreement will be adhered to, that Treasury Board Order 57 will continue to be applied and that any agreement reached between the parties will be honoured."

While the behind-the-scenes exchange of views was taking place between union headquarters and the ministry head office, the debate over the budget continued in the legislature. Grace McCarthy said, "I do want to assure those who are from the Kamloops area that it will be done well and with care, with the clients and those who live there being our very first priority." The correspondence demonstrated that the public arguments and the behind-the-scenes exchanges were continuing in a circular, never-ending stalemate.

Management said no meeting until the occupation ends, while the union said the occupation ends when government agrees to the contracts it had signed. The ministry then responded that it cannot commit to the contracts while the legislative future is uncertain, but they will consult when the occupation ends. And so on and so on, around it went.

Although it was true that the major reason for the government delay was the uncertain legislative future of Bills 2 and 3, there was another reason why the government was careful in both its public and private statements. Governments rarely put all their eggs in one basket in a labour relations dispute, and Bill Bennett's Social Credit government was no exception. While attempting to jam the legislation through, the government was quietly exploring the possibility of having the RCMP descend on the institution and arrest the union leaders in a move to restore order. When Jack asked Dave and me on the morning of July 20 if we had spoken to the RCMP, we did not know the extent of the discussions surrounding the possibility of a raid.

The RCMP had been criticized for decades as being the armed goons of employers during strikes, demonstrations and other confrontational tactics employed by the labour movement. Over the years, the RCMP repeatedly said they were not taking sides in so-called labour disputes, but to labour, the RCMP actions said otherwise. If mounties really were neutral, argued labour, why did the force always take management's side when there was a picket-line altercation?

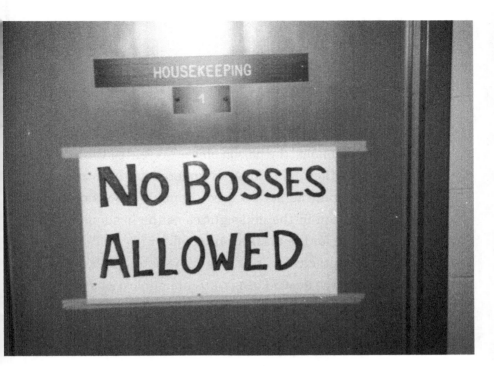

Another sign posted at Tranquille during the occupation. Gary Steeves

It was always striking workers who were arrested and charged even though managers and scabs were at least 50 percent responsible for issues on the line. Labour further criticized the force for not talking to unions. The RCMP made no effort to understand the issues the police were called upon to deal with.

In response to the criticisms from unions and central labour bodies like the BC Federation of Labour, the RCMP established an officer in their security service to act as liaison between unions and employers. The idea was to allow unions an opportunity, off the record, to discuss potential conflicts or other situations regarding RCMP conduct. It would also give mounties a heads-up to prevent police racing into situations armed only with management information and nightsticks. In the view of unions, the liaison officer prevented the RCMP from claiming they didn't know or understand the issues at hand. In general, the BCGEU used communications officer Robbie Robinson in the mid-eighties as the headquarters contact person for the RCMP's liaison officer.

Robbie contacted Jack Adams immediately after receiving a call from the RCMP. The BCGEU communications officer was used to getting quiet, off-the-record calls but this one surprised him. The RCMP labour liaison wanted to know what was really going on at Tranquille. Robbie's caller had alerted him to the fact that an element in the provincial government thought that using the police to stop the union occupation at Tranquille was a good idea and Robbie found out as much as he could before calling Jack immediately. Robbie was a charming operator. I liked him very much and learned a lot from him. He had a way of milking people for information and readily gathered facts before the person noticed how much they'd said to him. He had contacts galore and used them very strategically.

Robbie was hired by general secretary John Fryer when the union was expanding its staff and services. After the BCGEA under Norm Richards hired Fryer from the research department of the Canadian Labour Congress, Fryer inspired and led the evolution of the association into full union status. With a younger and more progressive provincial executive, the old association supported Fryer's drive for legal collective bargaining rights and the expansion of union benefits and services. As the union grew and matured, Fryer needed some professional specialists to help run it. Robbie was Fryer's choice to help craft and deliver the BCGEU message. Fryer recruited Robbie from the United Steelworkers District 6 office in Toronto. Robbie was working for Steelworkers District Director Bill Mahoney as a public relations specialist and was very happy to move to the west coast. Robbie soon put his wealth of experience to work for the BCGEU.

Robbie had an interesting background of experiences with the Steelworkers, an international union headquartered in Pittsburgh, Pennsylvania. While employed by the Steelworkers, Robbie had many training opportunities made available to him as a young communications specialist. Mahoney was by reputation a conservative union leader and a staunch anti-communist. He arranged for Robbie to take advantage of training opportunities outside of the union and one of those was the chance to attend a summer course in Langley, Virginia. The course was for communications operatives from the law enforcement and intelligence communities. This experience connected Robbie to other Canadians, many from the RCMP taking the CIA-developed-and-delivered course. Robbie had a million stories and a keen sense of humour, and he was not shy about sharing his stories with style and panache. Robbie was well connected with RCMP personnel and was never above contacting them if it met his need for information.

In recounting these events, I have used information that came directly to me from Robbie as well as some information that came directly to me from Jack Adams. I have checked with the BCGEU's legal counsel from 1983 and reviewed the cabinet documents from the same year and spoke to senior cabinet staff from that period. Although I will relate more on the review of cabinet documents later, neither our legal counsel nor the cabinet documents were of any assistance in shedding light on where the idea of the RCMP raid came from. There is no record I can find as to who took part in the discussions about such a raid. Senior cabinet staff speculated that cabinet discussions must have taken place, though they cannot recall any discussions being held. They further speculated that discussions around RCMP involvement were probably instigated by Norman Spector and/or Bob Plecas, senior officials in the premier's office.

Robbie Robinson shared his experience quite openly with me. His contact list in the RCMP had dwindled over the years, he said, but the BC division's labour liaison officer was a regular contact, especially when large strikes or demonstrations were in the offing. It was the labour liaison contact who alerted Robbie that the premier's office, through the attorney general's office, had made inquiries of the RCMP. The RCMP felt uncomfortable about responding with little information, so reached out to Robbie. True to his nature and instincts of acquiring as much information as he gave, Robbie wanted to know who had made the request but was never told. The RCMP officer outlined that the government said some union radicals had trespassed on government property and were obstructing government managers from carrying out their duties. Property and vulnerable human beings were at risk, and the police had to do something about it, preferably by arresting the union intruders. Robbie explained to the RCMP that resident care had not been affected, no property was disturbed or damaged in any way, and that the union's activity was being carried out by political activists not putschists.

Robbie argued effectively, as it turned out, that no laws had been broken and nobody's health and safety was in jeopardy. Further, it was the union members who worked at Tranquille carrying out the political protest. How would the RCMP look dragging middle-aged women away from their duties caring for people with developmental disabilities? Did the RCMP really want to get in the middle of the political fight between the union and the provincial government? From the conversation with his counterpart, Robbie got the feeling the RCMP did not want to get involved. Further, he got the impression from the liaison officer that the premier's office wanted the attorney general to order the RCMP to act.

When the RCMP informed their political masters that they preferred to stay out of the Tranquille situation unless serious criminal activity took place, government pushed back and asked the RCMP to reconsider. The RCMP, after all, was under contract with the BC provincial government to fulfill the role of BC's provincial police force. Robbie kept asking what laws were being broken, but the discussion always landed on trespassing.

The only people who were on the Tranquille property other than employees, residents and family members of Tranquille residents were Dave McPherson, me and two temporary BCGEU staff representatives: Diane Bird and Steve Wood. Arguably, Dave was there legally as he was the local staff representative handling grievances, which allowed access by advising management he would be on site. That left just me and two temporary union staff representatives. After Jack Adams' initial query, Dave and I quickly decided to send the temporary representatives back to the Kamloops office if legal confrontations were about to take place. The BCGEU used a temporary staff representative program to backfill regular staff positions that were vacant due to vacation, sick leave or pending hiring of permanent staff. The program took union activists off the job and assigned them union staff duties, usually in one of the union's twelve area offices. This gave local officers or shop stewards valuable experience handling grievances or other membership issues, and helped the union provide better services to its members. Most offices used some temporary support in the summertime especially. The local executive members and shop stewards chosen for temporary duties were carefully screened and placed on a pre-approved list for each area of the province.

Both Diane and Steve were on the pre-approved list and were extremely competent local officers. Diane was very intelligent, motivated and a capable leader who, in her everyday union life, was an administrative services local 1205 executive member.

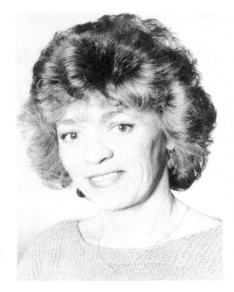

Diane Bird, BCGEU regional vice-president from Kamloops and a temporary staff representative who assisted with the occupation.
BCGEU Archives

Steve was chair of local 505, the retail stores and warehouse local representing liquor stores and the liquor distribution branch warehouse in Kamloops. He was tall and physically intimidating, but really just a teddy bear. Since Steve was with me most of the time in the first day or two of the occupation, it was a joke among us that Steve was my personal security guard. Steve's compassionate manner, quick wit and intelligent approach to problems contrasted to the jokes about personal security. Both Steve and Diane helped out in the initial days of the occupation, but returned to duties in the area office before the end of the occupation.

Robbie kept asking his RCMP contact if they thought arresting Diane, Steve and me would stop the occupation. How could the force stay out of the political dispute and engage in such arrests? How would dragging fifty-year-old female healthcare workers away in handcuffs aid the government's cause? As sensible as Robbie's points were, the back-and-forth between the RCMP and government officials went on for a couple of days. Eventually, the RCMP simply refused the government request on the grounds that no laws were being broken. Or at least that's what Robbie was told by his RCMP contact. The government was apparently not happy about the refusal, but Robbie, just doing his job helping the RCMP with information, had removed one large worry from the BCGEU leadership's list of concerns. If there were going to be legal issues to meet, they were not going to include criminal trespass charges laid by the RCMP.

It's possible that the RCMP made up the raid scenario in order to engage Robbie in a discussion of the Tranquille situation, but Robbie's detailed account suggests otherwise. If the desire to raid the occupation was real—and I believe it was—it must have been difficult for the government to accept the RCMP decision. Senior officials in the premier's office, by all accounts, hated the BCGEU. They saw the union as the enemy of the Social Credit government and the true opposition to Social Credit as a political party. Cabinet staff and former Social Credit MLA accounts of the government's ill will toward the union certainly explained the animosity that hung over every meeting and conversation between the government and the BCGEU. Political advice in 1983 from senior advisors like Norman Spector and Bob Plecas reflected the deep animosity they held for the BCGEU.

Jack Adams sounded very relieved that the RCMP was not going to be involved with the occupation action. Robbie joked with me on more than one occasion about how he saved me from jail. Other worries persisted, however, and they were more difficult to address. These other concerns were real and were given serious attention by union headquarters and the Tranquille locals. The most concerning among these issues required outside help to resolve. The help would come, but from unexpected sources. Residents of Tranquille had more friends than the union's leadership realized.

CHAPTER SEVEN

THE FEAR OF FAILURE

O ne overriding concern for the union, or at least for Dave and I, was the potential controversy around the death of a resident in the institution. Tranquille was an institution dealing with people who mostly required twenty-four-hour care. The vast majority of residents had significant developmental disabilities, and many had severe physical disabilities. Residents with more moderate disabilities were routinely placed in community living settings and replaced in the institution with people who had more challenging disabilities. In the twelve years prior to the occupation in 1983, an average of thirty-six Tranquille residents per year were placed in community settings after completing their education and training at the Tranquille institution.

New arrivals were typically more difficult to prepare for community placement. Most new admittances to Tranquille came from Woodlands School in New Westminster and were, in the words of the director of care, "more profoundly handicapped" due to similar patterns of placement and intake occurring at other institutions. We desperately needed individual placement plans (IPPs) for residents and fair treatment under Treasury Board Order 57 for employees. Those goals never changed throughout the occupation, and workers were firm in their belief that community placement without community services and resources in place would be disastrous for the residents they worked so hard to help.

Like all people, residents of provincial institutions do not live forever. But if a resident were to pass away during the occupation, the workers and their union would get the blame. Grace McCarthy would be viciously political and we knew it. Workers were merely standing up for their rights and the fair treatment of residents, but since a death was possible, we were forever mindful and fearful that a resident death would spark a government and public backlash from which we would never recover.

The best way to prevent our goals from being derailed was to demonstrate to the world how capable and caring staff at Tranquille were, and how well staff carried out their duties. Over the course of the occupation, we took a number of steps locally and provincially to provide comfort to anyone concerned about the quality of care residents were receiving. To reassure everyone that quality care for residents would continue, the members at Tranquille decided not to occupy the living wards of residents and the

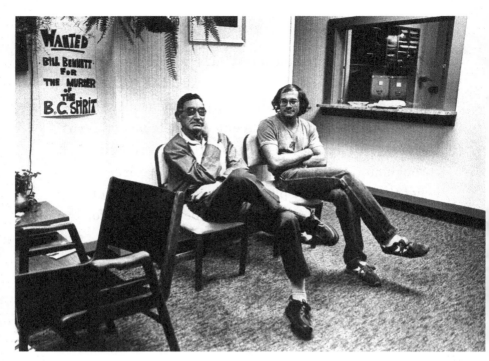

Union sentries "guarding" the main entrance to the administration building.

BCGEU Archives

union membership universally supported this decision. Leaving the living units alone was a wise decision on a number of levels. It meant that current arrangements for services to residents in their living quarters from outside providers such as doctors would continue as they were before the occupation. It meant management could check on conditions as usual, and saved union sentries from making a host of difficult decisions as various people came and went from these living areas.

Occupied buildings had restricted access. The restrictions applied to anyone other than union members from the BCGEU or the Union of Psychiatric Nurses (UPN). Sentries at doorways and indoor office entrances prevented non-union members from entering freely. The control of entry at main entrances required composure and patience as the constant flow of people in some buildings meant many judgment calls on the part of sentries. It also meant "old management" was ultimately prevented from entering any building except the living units of residents. Health care professionals and service providers periodically came and went but by not designating living wards as occupied sites, anyone, including a resident's visiting family members, could come and go as they pleased. It took a huge burden off the occupying union members, but the decision to leave living units and wards undesignated for occupation did not completely alleviate the fear of a care crisis.

Therefore, the BCGEU invited what may be called high-profile outsiders to visit and tour the facilities. These visits fit very well with the union membership's desire to educate the outside world on the important work they did with residents of the institution. The first high-profile visitor to the institution was Nelson Riis, member of parliament for Kamloops. Riis was a long-time resident of Kamloops, well known and well liked. His Robert Redford look-alike blond hair and good looks seemed to draw people to him. He had been a schoolteacher in the Kamloops public school system before taking a teaching position with Cariboo College. He served on Kamloops city council from 1973 to 1978, represented Kamloops on the board of the Thompson-Nicola Regional District and was a school trustee from 1978 until 1980. A fellow of the Royal Canadian Geographical Society, he stood for parliament in 1980 as a New Democrat and won 50 percent of the vote in the Kamloops riding. Four years later he captured 54 percent of the popular vote, beating his Conservative opponent by more than ten thousand votes.

A popular figure with demonstrated leadership skills, Riis was the perfect public figure to visit and comment on the state of affairs at Tranquille. The Riis visit occurred on Thursday, July 21. The media covering the union occupation were invited to accompany him and showed up in force. Riis was asked to provide his honest opinion of what he saw and how he felt things were being handled. The large contingent of media was asked to follow a couple of rules to protect the privacy of residents. No photos or use of names was allowed so that the residents' right to privacy would be respected. BCGEU members felt strongly that residents should not be used as props or pawns in the process of educating the public on the vital services employees provided. The visit of Nelson Riis was an overwhelming success. I do not know if Riis had ever been through Tranquille before, but the quality of care and the extensive services residents received clearly impressed him, and he said so.

The media was profoundly influenced by what they saw. For the first time, reporters could see for themselves what we were talking about. They saw the care needs of residents and the specialized training and treatment programs that staff delivered so professionally. The tone of the media coverage changed very quickly and Tranquille became the home of three hundred people rather than a government facility off in a remote corner of the Thompson River valley. Riis' complementary remarks about the staff and the state of affairs at the institution were music to our ears. Reporters who had accompanied Riis around the institution quickly corroborated his very positive assessment of the quality of care being provided.

John Fryer, now the president of our national union, the National Union of Provincial Government Employees (later to be renamed the National Union of Public and General Employees), visited on Thursday, July 27. BCGEU president Norm Richards addressed a membership meeting on Friday, August 5. These visitors could hardly be considered unbiased commentators on the conditions at Tranquille but they did generate media interest and of course boosted the morale of activists and members working at the institution. Bob Skelly, the NDP MLA from Alberni on Vancouver Island, was another visitor. Having prominent members of the legislature visit the institution helped both our educational efforts and the visibility of our protests at Tranquille.

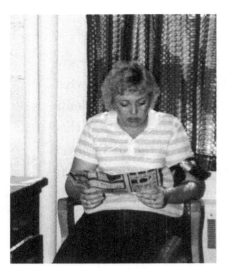

Erin Ireland, an occupation leader who conducted tours of the institution for journalists and other visitors. Gary Steeves

The most important visitors, however, were representatives of the British Columbia Association for the Mentally Retarded (BCAMR), the Kamloops Society for the Mentally Handicapped (KSMH) and the National Institute on Retardation (NIR). The organizations were effective advocates for the developmentally disabled and inherently suspicious of the BCGEU. The members of the BCGEU were equally leery of the advocacy organizations. The relationships between the organizations and the union were complicated and layered with misunderstandings and misconceptions. The BCAMR was in favour of deinstitutionalization and community living situations (primarily group homes) for institutional residents. The BCGEU thought the association was naive, being used by the government to save money.

Some elements of the union thought association members were profiteers more interested in operating their group homes to make a substantial living from the care of institutional residents. And in turn, the advocacy organizations believed the union was only interested in protecting the jobs of its institutional members, and increasing the wages and benefits of its members who were employed by the group homes. For example, employees of the Kamloops society were BCGEU members and very straightforward in their belief that they were undercompensated. The union, therefore, had treated many of the BCAMR member societies as employers bent on profit. Stories of inhumane care and exploitation were commonly exchanged and not nearly enough was done to understand the positions of the various players in life's complicated saga. The July 25 visit of David Vickers, president of the National Institute on Retardation and former deputy attorney-general, changed all that.

On July 2, the BC Association of Social Workers (BCASW) published a chronology pertaining to the proposed budget cuts to the Community Involvement Program (CIP). This program was to assist getting institutional residents into community settings. The chronology, entitled "Actions Taken Regarding Budget Cuts," noted the attempts by BCASW to convince the government of the folly of terminating the provincial government's important CIP for four thousand BC recipients. The scenario strongly indicated the government saw deinstitutionalization as a money-saving exercise. It reinforced the belief of critics that the BCAMR was being used in a strategy to save money, and the losers were going to be services to the developmentally disabled. Sometime in the frantic activity and madness unleashed by the July 7 budget and its accompanying legislation, BCGEU headquarters and David Vickers connected. At the Tranquille level, occupation leaders saw this was an opportunity to show the superior quality of programs they delivered and allay the fear that the ministry was peddling.

The July 25 visit was more than any of us could have hoped for. The ad hoc occupation committee had prepared a list of four things to be negotiated with management. On that list was the "establishment and complement of the resource/planning team" which David Vickers strongly endorsed. The BCGEU and the UPN saw the possibility of a partnership to force government into a bona fide placement process based on the needs of people, not the government. Vickers was accompanied by Elise Clark, past president of the BCAMR, and they held a news conference following the tour. Ironically, it was the same day that the MHR fired all its mental retardation coordinators province-wide.

Vickers and Clark stated their concern about the deinstitutionalization process, including the lack of individual placement plans for residents and the jobs of the Tranquille staff. They expressed the need for a "rational planning process" to ensure coordinated service delivery, standards of care and monitoring of services provided. Vickers and Clark agreed to cooperate with the BCGEU for the development of a closure plan that involved workers, parents, clients and their advocates. The union had gained a valuable ally in its fight to achieve justice for the residents, and I think the advocacy organizations felt the same about the union. The BCGEU issued a press release criticizing the government for not involving "unionized workers, local or provincial associations for the mentally retarded, parents, community groups, advocates or the unions themselves" in a process to guide government policy in a "more appropriate fashion." Arrangements were already in the works to build a broad and substantial policy group to put placement plans on a more comprehensive and professional footing.

On July 28, representatives of the BC Association for the Mentally Retarded, the Kamloops Society for the Mentally Handicapped, the BCGEU, the UPN and the new management at Tranquille, boarding home operators, the Kamloops School District, Cariboo College, homemakers and residents of Tranquille met at the Kamloops United Church Christian Education Centre. The purpose of the meeting was, in the words of the union, "to develop a plan to phase out Tranquille through a sane and rational process based on the needs of the residents rather than on the expediency of the provincial treasury." David Vickers chaired the meeting. The MHR was invited but did not show up. The group published extensive minutes under the title, "Community Planning and Resource Meeting," including the eleven principles agreed upon, the elements involved with a joint-planning process and next steps each organization would undertake. The commitments of the parties did seem very sincere and were reinforced on July 30 when the *Vancouver Sun* published an interview with Vickers. In the interview, the president of the National Institute on Retardation outlined the list of principles agreed upon by the July 28 meeting participants, including the following:

- a general service plan should be set up for each individual;
- there should be no shuffling of patients to other institutions or establishment of mini-institutions;
- standards of service should be established; and
- the government should make a commitment of adequate resources to do the job.

The new management committee at Tranquille met later on July 30 to discuss the July 28 Vickers meeting and agreed to assist with the planning process. The committee members were cautious but positive about the path forward. But perhaps the most passionate defence of the new-found opportunities for planning and the future care of residents was launched by Vickers himself in an interview with a Kamloops newspaper on August 2. The article entitled "Widgets yes, people no" began with Vickers "angrily responding to recent claims by the Kamloops Society for the Mentally Handicapped that the community can accept between eighty and a hundred of Tranquille's residents by the end of next year." Vickers said, "We're not talking widgets, we are talking people." The union and Tranquille members

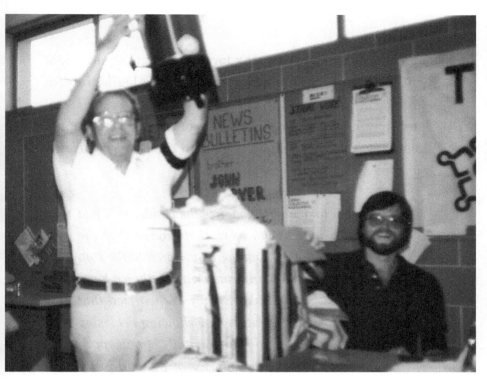

BCGEU Local 205 chairperson Bill Rhode wins first prize, a coffee pot, during "Fun Night" at Tranquille during the July–August 1983 occupation.

Gary Steeves

in particular were impressed with his understanding of the time constraints associated with preparing the move of so many individuals with acute and differing care needs.

The fear of failure had now dissipated. The union's strategy of outsiders touring the facilities and the building of understanding with interested parties and the media had succeeded. Media comments now reflected a deeper understanding and sympathy for the Tranquille situation. Jack Brooks of the *Vancouver Sun* quoted Alex McIntosh, director of nursing at Tranquille, as saying, "I have absolutely no concerns about the welfare of the residents." John Johnson's August 3 opinion column in the *Kamloops News* was typical. He said:

> *It isn't that to deinstitutionalize the residents is bad. The professionals who work there agree that the long-term goal of moving the residents into the community to live in more informal settings than a large institution is a good idea... They are worried that the haste the government is now showing in closing Tranquille, which is home to mentally handicapped people from all over the interior of BC, will prove disastrous for many of the residents, because they aren't and, perhaps more importantly, because the community isn't ready for them... the employees also wonder how McCarthy can talk about moving people into the community at the same time that workers whose job it is to coordinate the return of the mentally handicapped into the community are being fired.*

Johnson quoted healthcare worker Erin Ireland as saying, "the concerns for the residents come before any thought the employees are giving to their futures." The Johnson opinion piece concluded with the thought that when employees and resident advocates start talking, "the government should start answering their legitimate questions." The stage was now set for the unions to try and reach an agreement with the provincial government to accommodate the needs of the 325 residents as well as the 600 employees of Tranquille. Most interested parties, except the government, were on the same page and the BCGEU was prepared to take the lead. Our members demanded it.

Unbeknownst to the union, as the old Tranquille management listened with little or no interest in meaningful negotiations, the Kamloops Society for the Mentally Handicapped was meeting secretly with Grace McCarthy and her officials. Dan Meakes, the society's executive director, later told Dave McPherson that the minister offered to increase the society's funding from the ministry by six million dollars "to assist with transition." The ministry was clearly enticing the society to accept placement for another hundred Tranquille residents in the Kamloops area. Meakes related that the ministry would set up what he called a "tendering system" to expand group home operations in Kamloops. The ministry did not like the term "tender system" used to describe the expansion, but ministry officials made it clear that group-home operators were to submit bids to the ministry. Care of human beings was being tendered to the lowest bidder. So much for careful planning and individual placement based on care needs.

The information about the confidential meeting goes a long way to explaining David Vickers' strong statements in the Kamloops media the day before. He undoubtedly knew of the meeting between MHR and KSMH officials and its purpose. For me, it was just another example of the closure of institutions being about money and Social Credit manipulation. It was clear to the BCGEU leaders of the Tranquille occupation that much remained to be done. We had new allies. We had better-educated journalists and a better-educated public thanks to media coverage. We had a motivated membership prepared to try any tactics to get community care, and other transition issues on the negotiations agenda. But we had big troubles with the honesty and trustworthiness of government concerning Tranquille residents and their caregivers. So on August 4 we continued with our outreach, hosting a tour by the staff of group homes operated by the Kamloops Society for the Mentally Handicapped.

We had fully exposed, at least to ourselves, the government as a difficult, determined and devious adversary bent on achieving closure at all costs. Regardless of the government's attitude, the Tranquille workers were fearless and forged ahead. Union leaders and activists began to hold out some hope and optimism that we really could get something done for both employees and residents. The employee interests were likely to be dealt with at the big table, negotiating for all provincial government employees. Those negotiations were set to start in the fall, but the matter of the treatment of residents was now on the local table and positioned the union to at least try to move government on a more appropriate placement process. BCGEU members at Tranquille redoubled their efforts to continue the occupation, and to run the institution in an efficient and compassionate matter.

CHAPTER EIGHT

NEW MANAGEMENT OPERATIONS

T ranquille was a very large institution with a very complex operation. With 325 residents and 600 staff in who
knows how many departments on over sixteen hundred hec-
tares of property, setting up a governance structure was
challenging. The structure had to represent everyone and
all their departments and work units. I was working with a
subcommittee of the ad hoc occupation committee to
develop and recommend a democratic structure to serve the
union membership during the occupation. On July 24, the
ad hoc committee received and considered our recommendations for the creation of a new management committee.
Coincidentally, that afternoon the Union of Psychiatric
Nurses (UPN) had decided to officially join the occupation.
The formal decision was important, but it should be understood that the UPN membership had been fully involved in
the occupation prior to the formal decision. The UPN could
now be included in the formal governing structure and

receive the recognition they deserved for the tremendous efforts made by their members during the occupation.

The subcommittee I was working with proposed a new management committee with thirteen elected members and four ex-officio members. The committee would have a chair, three vice-chairs and nine executive members, each representing a department in

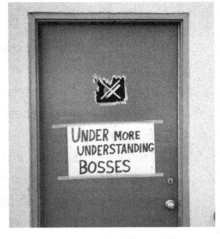

Another sign posted at Tranquille during the occupation. Gary Steeves

the institution including the Ministry of Agriculture and the BC Building Corporation. Each of the vice-chairs had a specific area of responsibility and, like the chair, would be elected at large by the membership. Each executive member would be elected from the department they represented. These department or work units were dietary; housekeeping; laundry; administration; social work and psychology; BC Building Corporation; healthcare workers; agriculture; and UPN. The ex-officio members would be me, Dave McPherson, Steve Wood and Terry Green. The BCGEU ex-officio members were permanent or temporary staff. The ad hoc committee accepted the structure and the recommendation to hold nominations and elections the next day, Monday, July 25 at the 8 p.m. membership meeting. Balloting would start at midnight and the new management committee would meet every night thereafter at 7 p.m. in the new BCGEU headquarters, formerly the conference room in the East Pavilion.

The elections generated intense interest. The ad hoc committee had decided that no further occupation-related actions would occur until after the election of the new management committee. There were, however, quite a number of acclamations including chair Bill Russell; vice-chair/community liaison Dawn Brookes; executive member-dietary Joch Copeland; executive member-laundry Linda Bruner; executive member-administration Marg Seagris; executive member-social work and psychology Kathe Freebury; executive member-BC Building Corporation (maintenance) Archie Brown; UPN's Doris Fesser; and Bob Lalonde, the executive member from the agriculture ministry. Following some hotly contested elections, the remaining new management committee members were chosen. Ian MacArthur was elected vice-chair for rostering; Janet Arnould, vice-chair for communications; Dave Boechler, executive member-housekeeping; and Pat Shtokalko, executive member representing healthcare workers. Pat defeated Erin Ireland, the tireless care worker who conducted tours and helped the media throng understand it was all about the humans living and working at Tranquille.

The establishment of a governing body was fundamentally important. Although the ad hoc committee had dealt with the initial arrangements and decisions regarding what the employees called "the sit-in," there were a spate of arrangements and issues to be attended to on a daily basis. A body with the confidence of the membership to decide on these day-to-day matters was an absolute necessity. By the evening of July 26, the new management committee was in full democratic management mode. The old excluded managers were really not needed other than to sign off on expenditures and reports necessary to keep the operation going. About one half hour per day was my calculation of how much time was required by old management.

The occupation of Tranquille buildings, based on ad hoc committee decisions and general membership meeting decisions, had taken the two main administration buildings on the night of the July 19 and had quickly moved to take control of the cafeteria complex the next day. The fire hall had been the fourth building to be secured by the union and that happened on the night of Thursday, July 21. Between the 21st and the 26th, the union banned management from five other departments or operation centres including the Centennial building (where housekeeping, stores, the pharmacy and staff lounge were located), BC Building Corporation (BCBC) maintenance facilities, the garage, the powerhouse and the laundry. Old management had been holed up in what was called the village office. The village was a community living simulation, an important part of the training program to prepare residents for living in the community. It had a small office and old management had used the village office periodically after their offices were occupied on the evening of July 19.

On July 26, old management's world changed again when the decision was made to occupy the office facility in the village as well as the carpentry offices and all Ministry of Agriculture buildings. These seizures meant that only the institution's residential wards were not occupied by the two Tranquille unions (BCGEU and UPN). Sentries and twenty-four-hour security was put in place to ensure an effective occupation. In a press release, I said, "the seizure of all non-ward facilities is now complete," noting that of the sixteen buildings at Tranquille, six were residential housing wards while the other ten were occupied by the union. There were nine "sit-in posts": the main administration building, the East Pavilion, the cafeteria, the fire hall, BCBC's shop, the laundry, the carpentry shop, the building maintenance shop and the village offices. These sit-in posts were sometimes quiet but more often than not were places where much socializing took place. Workers engaged in intense political discussions, played games (Trivial Pursuit anyone?), sang songs and wrote poetry. In many ways, these sit-in posts were where the real decisions about the occupation were made. Visiting these locations on evening strolls around the institution was always interesting and invigorating.

Old management was dispatched to a small cottage known as F-25 at the far end of the property and the main territorial protest was now complete. Not bad for just a week.

The new management committee issues, which were dealt with on a daily basis, fell into two general categories: health-care issues and physical plant and equipment maintenance issues. Meeting notes and agendas reflect the wide variety of matters that, in fact, took up most of the new management's meeting time. The agenda, after regular reports, began with a review of new business items. On July 26, for example, the new management committee dealt with the admission and discharge report, work orders for charge nurses, BCBC and the pharmacy, and the efficiency of the flow of mail. Although it toyed with issuing termination notices to the old manage-ment team, the new management committee stayed focused on practical business matters. For example, it resolved to replace the assistant laundry manager while vacation leave was being taken. Over the course of the occupation, the new management committee dealt with all manner of issues ran-ging from scheduling sentries, to letters to editors, MPs and MLAs, to serious questions of care.

One example of a question of care is worthy of note, as it was fairly typical of fundamental care issues the committee handled. The ministry denied the admission of a fourteen-year-old developmentally delayed client. The teenager's family required a break and needed respite care assistance. After a review of the ministry's emergency admissions policy, the union's new management committee decided to admit the youth. The committee found volume two, part two, para-graph I (a) of the ministry's own policy to be relevant and applicable to the situation of the fourteen-year-old: "The ministry's intent is to limit admissions to the aforementioned institutions (Woodlands, Tranquille and Glendale) to those children who require assessment only prior to a community or family placement, or for short-term respite care, or for behavioural management prior to a community or family placement." Reviewing and redesigning policy directives, maintaining accurate records of decisions, reviewing budget and managing communication issues was done routinely and professionally. For me, it was a wonderful group to work with. They made decisions quickly, accurately, efficiently and with the highest possible degree of sensitivity and empathy for residents and their families.

While the new management committee pondered the numerous operational issues on its agenda, BCGEU headquarters in Burnaby issued a scathing press release denouncing the MHR cuts to its programs. President Norm Richards called the cuts "a vicious attack by an anti-people government on the very old, the very young, the disabled and the poor." Decision-making duties continued as the new management committee worked hard to make the occupation effective and informative. It decided to restrict journalists' tours to one reporter at a time with no photos permitted. It granted a request by director of nursing Alex McIntosh to visit wards in the Village building. The permission was conditional on him calling the hotline to schedule an appointment, as anyone else would otherwise be required

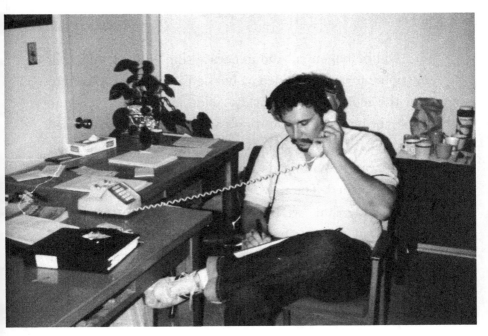

Steve Wood in "BCGEU Headquarters" at Tranquille during the occupation.

Gary Steeves

to do, and be accompanied by a senior member of the new management committee. The work of the committee continued much the same each day. One exception occurred on July 27 when old management somehow intercepted the paycheques for employees of the institution. Steve Wood intervened, however, and the cheques were distributed in the usual fashion, much to the satisfaction and relief of staff. More typical of the new management committee was the July 29 decision to move a band concert for residents, originally scheduled for September, up to the first week of August.

Old management did generate some issues, which in my opinion were intended to hassle the workers' efforts to run the institution smoothly. Aside from the paycheque issue, the building corporation's old management expressed concerns at the level of service the new management committee was providing as far as fire protection services were concerned. The new management committee replied immediately that "we have extra patrols, one extra man per shift at no pay and an understanding that the chief will participate if there is a fire." New management further pointed out that these arrangements and regular checks of equipment are "all in addition to the normal high level of service." Old management either made a mistake or were playing games to try and remain relevant. But the workers and their new management committee were so far ahead of the handful of overpaid and underworked old managers on care and maintenance issues that nothing except learning opportunities came of the old management games. And ironically, when the fire chief was absent for a period, new management had to impose existing policy and procedures on the building corporation to fill the temporary vacancy.

Senior managers, in my opinion, did not seem to be needed. The workers of Tranquille could run that institution with professional efficiency and skill, which seemed part of the culture of the place. And the workers were simply exemplary. As the new management committee and the ex-officio union officials (mainly Dave and me) tried to keep the focus on the important work Tranquille does and its impact on residents and communities, old management would make another mistake. One example was the August 1 presentation the union and new management had prepared for Kamloops city council. It was detailed and informative but a series of screw-ups by old management involving a family visiting a resident diverted attention to the human care issues they raised.

Cottage F-25 had been booked for the Prince George family of a Tranquille resident, but old management refused to move as they were using it for an office. The cottage was one of five or so available for visiting families and old management could have easily used another cottage. The family had to be put up in a local motel, which the ministry paid for. This situation upset some staff and outright angered others. The new management committee discussed the matter at length and took action. New management decided to occupy the cottage, thereby kicking old management out and making it available for use. I was quoted in the *Kamloops Daily Sentinel* on Tuesday August 2 explaining, "We occupied the house (cottage F-25) to stop management from playing games with plans and schedules. We will make the house available to the next family supposed to use it." I could not resist adding, "the place runs as smooth and in many cases a hell of a lot better without them."

There was one time when human care issues collided with the physical plant and equipment maintenance issues.

It was serious and demonstrated the attitude of old management and MHR, as well as the courage and determination of the workers at Tranquille. Early in the occupation I had met with our members in the BC Building Corporation (BCBC) maintenance operation and asked what the procedure was for fixing things around the institution. I used a broken doorknob as an example. They said that if they saw a broken doorknob or anything else that needed attention, they would report it to their foreman (who was in the union) and he would give it to the boss. The boss would fill out a work order determining when he wanted it done, and give it to the foremen who would then schedule a maintenance person to do the work. They complained it took weeks to change a light bulb sometimes.

I suggested we change the procedure. They agreed and made a suggestion of their own. If a maintenance person saw something that needed fixing, they would just fix it. That would be the new policy. The foremen could fill out the paperwork after the work was done, give it to me and I would have old management sign the necessary form after the fact. The workers loved it, I thought it made sense, and the institutional staff appreciated things getting immediate attention. The medical records staff came to me to say thanks for getting their door fixed as they had been after old management for months to get the problem addressed.

The new procedure was blessed by the ad hoc committee and old management didn't blink in the morning when I

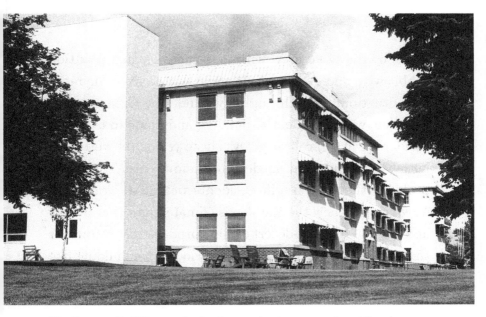

The Greaves Building cerebral palsy ward, where we replaced the air conditioning system. BCGEU Archives

took a pile of paper to them to sign, but the medical records door was not the only thing old management put off. I cannot be exactly certain of the date, but I think it was a Saturday. It was the first night I was not sleeping on the floor of our makeshift office in the East Pavilion. I was in a hotel room in downtown Kamloops when the phone rang around 9 p.m. or so. It was the BCBC foreman in a near state of alarm. The air conditioning unit on the roof of the Greaves building had given out.

I said, "Well can't your crew fix it?" and he replied no. He explained that the machine was old and had been kept going by the BCBC crew with extreme care and attention, rabbit wire and good luck. It could not be fixed anymore. The situation raced through my mind. The Greaves ward, so-called, was a residential building and home to over fifty residents with cerebral palsy. These residents were frail, largely immobile and needed continuous care. They were probably the most fragile residents we had at Tranquille. Anyone who knew the Kamloops climate knew that in July and August, the high-desert climate produced temperatures that were inhumanely hot. An old wood-frame building like the Greaves building would, without air conditioning, heat to a level unfit for human habitation. Moving the residents was unthinkable, so replacing the unit was our only option.

The BCBC crew chief said that they had been recommending a new unit for a few years, but old management had not approved purchase and installation. Two years ago, however, the cost of a new unit was put in the budget and approved. Old management had ordered a new unit but never paid for it. The huge rooftop unit was stored in a Kamloops warehouse as the ministry had never proceeded with installation. In short, there was a new unit in Kamloops and the budget for it was approved. This new unit would have to be retrieved from the warehouse, loaded on a flatbed truck, transported to Tranquille from the warehouse, unloaded with a crane and placed on the roof of the Greaves building. The old unit would have to be removed by crane and disposed of in the usual manner. BCBC maintenance workers could hook up the new unit to the existing pipes and connections, and with luck, cool air would flow. And all this would have to be done before the heat of the morning sun took its toll on our Greaves residents and staff.

"Can it be done?" I asked. To my great surprise, the crew chief said it could. He would have to get some people out of bed and work all night, but it was possible. I knew I would have to get old management to sign off on the bill after the fact so the supplier would get paid, but it needed to be done and by the time I got there in the morning, it was. Our BCBC members and the truck and crane operators were amazing. Their dedication said it all to me. I was so happy to feel cool air coming out of the system. The continued operation of the Greaves ward in comfortable temperatures was a testament to the commitment of care the workers had for Tranquille residents.

A couple days later I got the paperwork to take to Terry Prysiazniuk and the old management team in a cottage at the back of the property. Everyone knew the huge bill for the rooftop air conditioning unit was in the file. I opened the file and was shocked at the six-figure bill. I am embarrassed to admit that I cannot remember the exact amount, but it was a lot. The cost of the unit, the cost of the truck and crane, the storage fees, miscellaneous supplies, accessory materials and overtime all around, I think, added up to about $100,000. The secretary in the admin office asked if I wanted it on the top or the bottom of the pile of documents to be signed. Jokingly, I said to hide it in the middle. But there was no hiding it; everyone wished me luck as I proceeded to meet with the ministry's old management. Dave McPherson and a small group of new management and media were ready to join us. I had arranged with Dave that if I gave him a signal, he would bring the media scrum to Terry and I to witness the debate over whether the expense bills should be signed off.

Terry and I went to an old picnic table outside the cottage. He signed a number of papers and then came to the substantial BCBC wage bill. When he saw the rooftop air conditioning unit bill, he dropped the papers and said, "I'm not signing this." I explained the situation we'd faced and told him he had better sign. He refused, mumbled about authority and special permissions and I interrupted him. "So you would just let the Greaves residents die," I said. He looked at me half angry, half puzzled. I said something to the effect that if he did not sign, he and I were going to talk to the media, and he could explain why he and the ministry were prepared to let residents die for the sake of money.

He looked deflated and defiant all at once. He grabbed the paper and signed the documents and dropped them on the table as if they were as hot as the Greaves ward in the summer sun. I tried to hide my relief and quickly left for the awaiting new management committee. I tried to not yell, skip, cartwheel or otherwise display my relief and delight as I carried the folder of signed documents across the field toward Dave and the others. Everyone was relieved and smiling as one of the admin office staff said to me, "Well I guess we can do anything. What about a new roof?"

Just five days before the occupation ended (August 7 or 8, I believe), the new management committee found a budget allocation to pay $92,000 to upgrade a van to accommodate wheelchairs or purchase a new van if upgrades were not possible. On July 30 the *Vancouver Sun* reported that "almost $1.5 million worth of renovations are continuing at Tranquille Centre for the Mentally Handicapped even though the institution is scheduled for closure by the end of next year." Maurice Cownden, corporate affairs manager for the BC Building Corporation, confirmed a new sprinkler system, fire alarms and fire exits were expected to be finished by November 1983.

Did Terry Prysiazniuk know about the BCBC work plans? Hard to believe he didn't. Was he playing games with me as he agonized over signing the bills? Was BCBC really more concerned about fire doors than the livability of their residences in stifling summer heat? The audacity of the MHR and the BCBC to ignore human needs and throw money at the protection of their property was revealing for me. It was even more revealing to see the dilapidated state of the building in 2019 still standing and unused since the closure three and a half decades earlier. There's no question that the government did not get their money back on those expenditures.

The more I learned about the Tranquille closure, the lower my opinion became of Grace McCarthy and her ministry. There was no indication they cared about the people for whom they were responsible. It was all about money while the workers, on the other hand, displayed a highly competent, creative and motivated character. It was no wonder Tranquille workers were offended by the treatment they received from their employer, but the new management committee continued in its day-to-day struggle to oppose the government's inadequate plans.

CHAPTER NINE

SONGS, POETRY AND PROTEST

As my friend Dave MacKinnon used to say to me, "every campaign, every social movement, every strike or social protest has its own music and artists performing for its cause." That certainly was true in the American civil rights movement, the anti-war protests over Vietnam and the other social upheavals of the 1960s. MacKinnon even asserted that one cannot have a bona fide protest movement without music and art as popular features of the struggle. Carlos Santana was more to the point. He said, "When you play music, you bring light into the darkness." Tranquille and its staff certainly deserved more light, and fortunately it was there, awaiting an opportunity to shine.

On July 21, after a hectic forty-eight hours of building occupations, media scrums and generally reorganizing everyone's life, an evening union membership meeting was being held in the cafeteria. It was rather chaotic with different groups and departments talking amongst themselves.

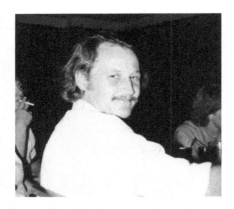

Dave McPherson on August 9, 1983, the day the occupation ended.

Gary Steeves

Logistical issues were being sorted out and various matters were dealt with by those affected as they arose. Debbie Forehead, a twenty-year-old auxiliary healthcare worker approached Dave McPherson and me as we sat at the front of the cafeteria. Years later she admitted to me that she was nervous. On July 20 she had worked a regular shift and came back to join the occupation. After introducing herself to Dave and me, she talked about how she found eating and sleeping in a rather communal fashion fascinating, and felt that everything we did during the occupation was more about the residents than the employees. And that, she said, was important to her.

She also told us she had written a song. In fact, she had written three, but she was ready to sing her first one now. She was totally taken aback when I said, "Oh good. Sing it." She had expected us to take her to a separate room, but now she found herself performing in front of a few hundred Tranquille staff. She opened her guitar case as Dave called everyone to order. She played beautifully and sang unbelievably well. The song started:

The rain began in the spring of 1983
when on May 5 they signed a death warrant for BC

and went on:

> *No taxes they told us are gonna go up, you just wait*
> *   and see*
> *so we waited—now it's hell for you and me*
> *Then summer came and brought no sun and the*
> *   budget was announced*
> *but the words we heard weren't what we hoped for,*
> *   dictatorship was pronounced*
> *The doctor's bill came yesterday, not covered by*
> *   Medicare*
> *'cause our right to healthcare is no longer there*
> *A letter came addressed to me, the paper inside was*
> *   pink*
> *and human rights were crossed out in blood not ink*

Thankfully, the chorus lifted everyone:

> *A roar arose across the land in 1983*
> *'cause the bill that promised everything forgot democracy*
> *and the people they were crying out "What can we do?"*
> *and as they spoke they pushed the legislation through*
> *A roar arose across the land in 1983*

A roar arose in the cafeteria as Debbie finished singing. Dave was on the phone immediately to CKNL, the local radio station. We hustled Debbie into a car and off we went to the NL studios and recorded the song. NL played it first as a news item, referring to it as the "anthem for Operation Solidarity." Local Kamloops media had always tied the occupation of Tranquille to the Operation Solidarity and Solidarity Coalition opposition movement.

Debbie Forehead (later Patten) was the daughter of English immigrants. In 1966, her father, mother and two kids left England where their living conditions were desperate. They settled in the Lower Mainland of BC where her father found work at the Oakalla Prison Farm. He subsequently went to work for Canadian Pacific Airlines while her mother found work as a secretary. They bought a house in Delta and two years later moved to Kamloops. The recession of the eighties took a toll on the family. As an auxiliary healthcare worker, Debbie was unable to financially assist either parent. Now she was facing job loss herself in a city with a 20 percent unemployment rate. She understood hardship, but she also understood the need to care for those less fortunate. All her life experience showed through in her songs. Debbie released her second song on the July 23:

I'm a union member, who wants Gracie's tenure
I'd show her what freedom means

Afraid of a police state where people don't rate
and money is master of all...

The song reflected the general feeling of Tranquille union members that big money and power were calling the shots and no one in power cared about those who could not care for themselves. Those that worked in the care field and the unions that represented caregivers had to stand up to the money and power because, as Debbie Patten said in an interview thirty-five years later, "If they didn't, who would?" Tranquille employees believed that if they could just talk to Gracie, the minister would see the value of their work as caregivers. As minister responsible for Tranquille, McCarthy could change government plans and redefine Tranquille's role in a more humane system of care for people with mental disabilities. The second verse of Debbie's second song got to that point:

We want security and not UIC
and welfare is not for us
so get off your tushes and come out of the bushes
please Gracie come talk to us

The BC Federation of Labour was impressed with Debbie's music and invited her to perform at the huge rally being planned for Empire Stadium on August 10. It was exciting news and Deb *did* perform at the giant protest.

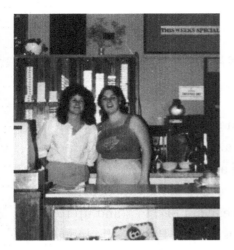

Debbie Forehead (right) in the Tranquille cafeteria during the occupation. Gary Steeves

Some of our union members at Tranquille were not particularly musical but many wrote their own stories, poetry and/or letters to make their feelings, their message and their opinions heard. Some were written to motivate fellow workers, like the anonymous poem "The Missing Element" in the July 23 edition of *Tranquille Tough Times*:

I.
There's a clever young fellow named SOMEONE ELSE,
There's nothing that person can't do,
He's busy from morning to way at night,
Just substituting for you.

2.
You are asked to do things to help yourself.
And you come back with a ready reply;
"Get SOMEBODY ELSE,
He'll do much better than I."

3.

There is so much to do in our union,
So much, and the workers are few,
SOMEBODY ELSE *is getting weary and worn,*
Just substituting for you.

4.

Right now we've got a struggle,
And the fight will be tough and long,
The Socreds want our freedom and rights,
But we'll fight back, learning to be strong.

5.

So the next time you're asked to do something,
Give me an honest reply,
"If somebody else can give time and support,
You can bet your last dime, so will I."

Tranquille Tough Times carried many clever pieces, which made daily reading entertaining and engaging. Some poetry recorded the political events and the circumstances of the budget, the proposed legislation and the occupation. *Tranquille Tough Times* carried a poem by "Just Passing Time" on August 2 that did just that, entitled, "TRANQUILLE OCCUPATION-AL THERAPY" or "EVERYTHING YOU WANTED TO KNOW ABOUT SITTING-IN BUT WERE AFRAID TO ASK." It read:

It's been fourteen days, let's not forget the nights
Morale is high, in our fight for human rights
While sitting in, we've made new friends
Which will endure when our occupation ends

Our building count is on the rise
You should hear our administrators sighs
Life as a nomad is not much fun
We'll all be glad when our job is done

There's twenty-four hours in our day
Though we only draw eight hours pay
It's no big deal we all want to stay
To show the province of BC the way

After a couple more verses, the author concludes with "The end of this poem is very near. We will be victorious, have no fear. Our stand will be remembered for many a year. So let's not forget why we are here." Four days before the end of the occupation, on August 5, "Dead and Tired" wrote another perspective with "A Sit-in's Prayer":

Help me, help me
Someone please
The bags 'neath my eyes
Are down to my knees.

The caffeine is running
Free through my veins
And my bodily strength
Steadily wanes.

The coffee is fine
If you don't add cream
Because if you do
It turns bright green.

My age lines have started
My hair's turning grey
Where's my relief?
Someone show them the way.

Three more verses lead to the final verse:

But it's not all that bad
This sit-in of mine
And if we all work together
We'll be doing just fine.

The *Tough Times* provided a unique opportunity to write to fellow protesters and the world. Some members contributed regularly and some were shy, choosing not to use their real names. But the poetry and prose that went into the *Tough Times* clearly showed that workers took ownership of their actions and were determined in their efforts. The union members from both the BCGEU and the UPN were extremely loyal to each other and those they cared for. They understood who was responsible for the situation at Tranquille and in the province, and they were determined to do their part to support each other and the residents of the institution. Some workers wrote serious critiques of the events of the day while others used humour to contribute. An August 3 piece entitled, "The Lord Giveth and Bennett Taketh Away," provided a little of both. It read:

> *I asked Bennett, "What have you to offer me?" And his answer came, "What have you to give?"*

> *You know you're in trouble when...*
> *...you know all the answers in Trivial Pursuit*
> *...you went to sleep in the cafeteria and woke up in the laundry*
> *... someone tells you the coffee you are drinking has been here since day one*
> *... people giggle when they tell you, "You talk in your sleep"*

> *Happiness is...*
> *... going to the canteen and they finally have your brand of cigarettes*
> *... finding an extra unoccupied green foamie*

... Grace McCarthy saying "I give in"
... Being told by the hotline there is lots of coverage
... a fresh pot of coffee.

The *Tough Times* published puzzles and games such as the August 4 "Fill in the Word" game which kept the people at the sit-in posts entertained for hours. The workers' determination was always on display, even as the occupation stretched into its third week. On August 6, just three days before the end and under the headline, "HUMOUR SHEETS," the *Tough Times* asked, "Why does the provincial government use Learjets and limousines to move garbage around??" finishing with a memo to Premier Bennett:

To Mr. Bennett & Company
  We do not want your crumbs i.e. "seniority back."
We want the whole loaf. Remove your July 7th legislation—then remove yourself.

Perhaps the best summary of the Tranquille situation in the most creative style was Ron Anderson's, "The Parable of Tranquille," published in the *Tough Times* on August 7, 1983:

And it came to pass that she with the red hair and forked tongue spoke from her high place in the inner sanctorium. Close that which is known as Tranquille and cast out those who abide there and yea even those who toil in that place. I know nothing of their plight or sickness but my gold shall be saved for much lesser things. That place shall be sold be it even unto my neighbour who is called A.G.

But it is written that they who abide within the walls of Tranquille could not speak for themselves even they who held great rank in that place would not utter on their behalf for they were under the spell of the red-headed one, but not so they that attended those human beings for they uttered a loud cry heard across the great land and even beyond for they saw the injustice in the red-headed one's words and great anguish came upon them. They that cared cast out those of high rank and took upon themselves the protection of the unfortunates so that she with the red hair and forked tongue would come to understand the plight of those who cannot protect themselves.

And it is said that the red-headed one's king who it is now known across this land to have yet a larger forked tongue and a five o'clock shadow at high noon, has told her to watch her step lest the ivory tower where they abide might fall upon them and then others with greater compassion for those who cannot help themselves will take their place.

But it is written that all should be wary of crumbs cast upon the land for crumbs do not a meal make. Therefore, accept only the whole loaf that all may enjoy the protection and peace long fought for by those that have gone before.

And so I say unto you, go ye into your village town or great city, enrich yourselves by joining the local society for the retarded and by your numbers cast out those that hear only the jingle of gold and rank put in their place those who are of understanding and compassion and let the red-headed one know that the promises made are null and void for this is the way to go for the protection of those for whom we care.

– Ron Anderson

A small unsigned poem followed Ron's parable. It reinforced the workers' notion of the need to respect the rights of all and complemented their union. It read:

Now there's Bill, hear what he's saying
The people are mad because of the jobs he's slaying
Well Gracey's got heart, though the budget is tight
She's abolished the human right.

But don't you worry, and don't you quit
Cause the fightin's not quite over yet
We're gonna rally and we're gonna sit
We've got the best union you've ever met.

The poems, the songs and the creative expression of Tranquille workers said it all. The last poem was published the day before the decision was made to end the occupation. The creativity of Tranquille workers, however, never ended. The collection of workers' artistic expression in the *Tough Times* provides a broad and deep cross section of emotion for the time and events in which they were engaged. And Deb's third song was lyrically the summary of the whole story. It went as follows:

We will march to make Bill see
The error of his ways
We are the people of BC
His party has betrayed

He'll take this province for his own
His name is Premier Bill
He'll take your job and home away
Your freedoms he will kill.

Chorus:

So Billy if you look around
You won't like what you see
We're fighting for democracy
Through Solidarity.

He's got the right to rule the land
It came in early May
But we'll march the streets from dawn to dusk
To make him see our way.

He doesn't care what cost it brings
The powerless will pay
He's hell-bound for restraint, my friend
Until our dying days

The pain is not the cost he knows
In dollars with no sense
He'll cut the public service by 25 percent.

We speak for those who have been touched
By Billy's master plan
The weak, the young, the elderly
The workers of this land.

He does things the way he likes
He has a majority
He'll take away your human rights
Your civil liberties.

He'll never break the fighting hearts
Of those he chose to wrong
We've got the strength to carry on

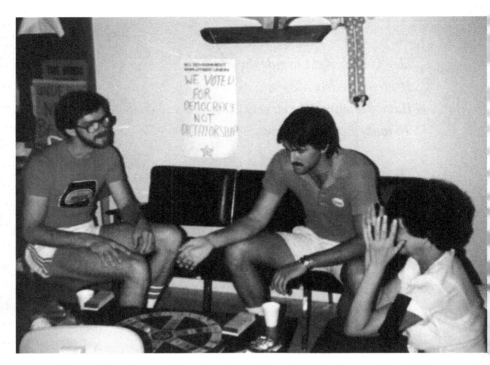

Tranquille union members play Trivial Pursuit during "occupation shift" at their workplace. Gary Steeves

Long after he is gone.

And when it comes his time again
We'll remember '83
We'll vote him down and kick him out
And restore democracy.

Negotiations with management had begun in earnest but the workers knew the fight was far from over. A difficult strike over worker's rights loomed ahead for the fall of 1983, but no one seemed worried or down. The workers at Tranquille were resilient and optimistic. They were simply a marvellous group of people who made a good union and deserved a better employer. MacKinnon and Santana were probably right because Tranquille workers did create the art for their movement and brought light to BC in '83. Negotiations over the future of the Tranquille residents were very much in the hands of the occupying forces and their new-found allies. A hard bargain was about to be made with potentially significant results for residents, families, advocates and workers.

CHAPTER TEN

NEGOTIATIONS AND DE-OCCUPATION

From the very start of the occupation on July 19, everyone knew that it would end one day. No one, including Dave and me, had any idea how the occupation would turn out, but we knew what we wanted to happen. Or at least we thought we knew. We knew we could put pressure on the government. We knew we could focus public criticism on the budget and its twenty-six bills. We knew we could expose the government's agenda, and we hoped to make a difference for the residents at risk in the process. The glare of public attention needed to shine on the government's mean-spirited and dishonest agenda. Unions always look for innovative ways to inform their members and negotiate solutions to their problems. We knew the occupation would have an educational impact on people, especially those who had no idea what Tranquille did, and we knew we would have to negotiate an end to it.

How far the occupation would have to go to achieve its goals was anyone's guess on July 19. One of the obvious challenges for the labour movement in its fight against the budget was the length of time until their collective agreements expired. Public sector unions were the most directly affected by Bills 2 and 3, which aimed to eliminate any meaningful protection for public sector workers. The BCGEU agreements expired November 1, 1983. The question of how unions could maintain an effective opposition campaign from the beginning of summer until the end of October was very real.

The NDP opposition was waging an effective battle in the legislature against the Socreds' twenty-four-hour legislation by exhaustion. Endless debate and filibuster slowed progress, but there were limits to stopping a majority government who could use closure to ram bills through. Unions and community allies did everything they could to oppose the government's intentions. They organized rallies and other public events designed to educate and organize opposition. They used every conceivable method to display public displeasure with what the government was doing, and unions pushed the legal limits by engaging in various job actions and wildcat strikes. In the Kamloops area, for example, there were sixteen job actions including seven wildcat strikes from the beginning of the occupation on July 19 until August 6. The Tranquille occupation helped

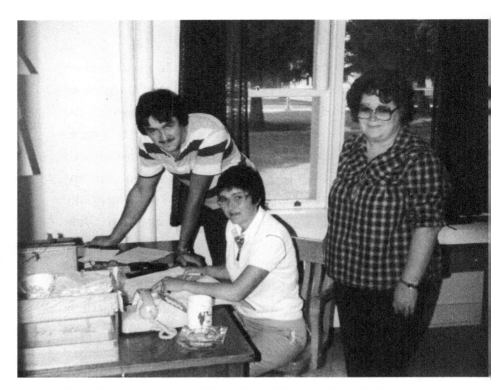

Dawn Brookes (seated) and Janet Arnould in the hotline/scheduling centre. It operated twenty-four hours per day. Gary Steeves

buy valuable time for opposition forces to organize and defy the government's legislative agenda.

The occupation also provided inspiration that a fight back was possible. Dozens and dozens of unions and labour organizations sent telexes and telegrams of encouragement to Tranquille workers and many noted the inspirational effect the occupation was having on their members. These unions covered the full spectrum of public and private sector as well as BC Federation of Labour affiliates and non-affiliates. In hindsight, I wish we had worked the media more astutely, but the unknown nature of the occupation's scope and duration, and the need to manage the occupation and negotiate outcomes worked against us doing more than we did with the media. After all, unions are all about negotiations and successful bargaining is real work requiring patience, attention to detail and a clear vision of what you need.

Fortunately, our negotiations were quarterbacked by one of the best: Cliff Andstein. Negotiations had started in a low-key manner via the July 20 letter from John Noble to Norm Richards. Cliff and I had discussed the approach I should take with local management later that day. According to my notes of the discussion with Cliff, we developed five fundamental questions to pose:

1. Has MHR established a planned process for residents?
2. When does planned process start?
3. Will Treasury Board Order 57 apply regardless of Bills 2 and 3, as well as current provisions of the collective agreement?
4. How many jobs are available in the public service outside Tranquille?
5. How will public service jobs be offered to displaced workers? When?

Cliff advised me that he would respond to Noble and he did so on Thursday, July 21. The reply to the deputy minister got right to the point. It said that management had noted "an air of uncertainty due to the pending legislation," and asked if that meant the MHR would wait until legislation was passed and the collective agreements nullified before it addressed employees of the institution. "Our members at Tranquille want a written commitment from the minister that the provisions of the collective agreement will be adhered to, that Treasury Board Order 57 will continue to be applied, and that any agreement reached between the parties will be honoured." The letter ended with, "I personally fail to understand why your minister will not agree to honour those previously reached agreements."

In hindsight, a walk-through of the cabinet documents that have now been publicly disclosed from 1982 and 1983 sheds light on that issue. The arbitrary 25-percent across-the-board staff cuts that the cabinet authorized and directed in 1982 could not be realized in the MHR without the closure of a large institution. Cliff Andstein intuitively understood what was going on. He was an experienced negotiator, and a well educated and intelligent leader in BC's labour movement. I could not have asked for a better director to work with and we became good friends. Like me, Cliff was from New Brunswick. He had moved west, got an education and was working as an instructor at the BC Institute of Technology when John Fryer hired him to the BCGEU. Fryer was quickly assembling a talented team of young and motivated staff to organize, negotiate and arbitrate the provincial government into the twentieth century.

When the MHR negotiations over Tranquille started, Cliff was overseeing the unknown. Accompanied by Dave McPherson, Steve Wood and Dan Hales, I went off to a meeting with local managers Terry Prysiazniuk, Gord Begley, Brent Johnson and Alex McIntosh. I put to them the questions Cliff and I had discussed that morning. Is there a planned process in place, when does it start, how many jobs are available and how many Tranquille employees would qualify? We also asked for a written commitment regarding the collective agreement and Treasury Board Order 57. Management had little to say. They advised us that they would have to contact Victoria and get back to us. No progress locally, but the response came to union headquarters by way of a letter to President Richards.

Cliff telexed the content of the letter to me and it clearly showed the ministry was completely unprepared for the union actions and questions. It said, "We are in the process of developing our plans." Condescendingly, Noble added, "My staff will be pleased to discuss implementation with you." Noble also offered consultation with the union "providing you cease the disruption of operations at Tranquille." I suspect Minister McCarthy imposed this condition to cease occupation on her deputy and other ministry officials; we would hear it constantly for the next couple weeks.

Noble's Friday, July 22 letter to Richards made two additional points that were central to understanding the government's intentions. First, he said, "I can make no statement whatsoever with respect to matters before the legislature. It is the intent of government, however, to develop the compensation package for employees... You are encouraged to submit your recommendations regarding such compensation provisions." There was every indication that they had no intention of negotiating anything with the union, completely consistent with the union's legal analysis of Bill 2. Noble arrogantly concluded the letter with, "I await your response to my request for consultation and for your agreement to cease interference with the management of the operations of Tranquille."

Noble's letter was sent by telex at 1 p.m. on Friday the twenty-second. At 2:22 p.m., the union responded by saying, "The union is in receipt of your initial proposal regarding the closure of Tranquille Hospital. This proposal is vague and leaves many questions unanswered. However, a union committee is prepared to meet with you at a mutually agreeable time and place to continue negotiations in an effort to achieve a settlement." The letter, drafted by Cliff, concluded with a reminder that there was currently a collective agreement and a Treasury Board Order in place that contain a compensation package for affected employees. The effort to ignore the ministry's paternalism and maintain a relationship based on a "bargaining relationship of equals" was masterful.

The ministry continued with plans to axe 345 ministry employees across BC before it would deliver a similar fate to 600 Tranquille employees. On Monday, July 25, when union headquarters levelled a blistering criticism of the government's service cuts and condemned the termination of hundreds of BCGEU members, the occupying forces at Tranquille tightened their control of the institution. As negotiations stalled, our new management committee began to hype the Empire Stadium rally in Vancouver as the culmination of the protest phase of Operation Solidarity. It also increased its efforts to coordinate a flood of letters to newspaper editors from Tranquille workers.

In the background, the negotiations committee worked on a package that could end the occupation. From the July 22 meeting with management until early August, the occupation continued to tighten its control of the institution and fine-tune what it felt was acceptable in terms of a de-occupation agreement. Subtle messaging was exchanged between the union and the ministry, but it was not until Monday, August 1 that a face-to-face meeting was contemplated. Eventually, August 3 was set for the meeting between the new management's negotiations committee and Tranquille management.

The general agreement that the negotiations committee, Dave McPherson and I had drafted included:

1. an amnesty agreement from the appropriate ministries and the BC Building Corporation;
2. the establishment of a resource planning team to guide placement of residents;
3. a labour/management committee to oversee employee transition; and
4. the retention of a BCGEU office on the Tranquille premises.

As an aside, the union offered to pay for any expenses associated with operating an office on the premises. The important part of the package was the resource planning team with BCGEU social workers, dieticians, therapists, care aides and UPN nurses, as well as David Vickers and other advocates and family members. BCGEU activists believed that such a multidisciplinary team would improve the community placement project. The amnesty agreement was the same sort of agreement used by unions and management as part of the settlement of a strike: "It is therefore agreed by the Parties to this agreement that no intimidation, harassment, discrimination, discharge, nor any other form of disciplinary action shall be taken against a union member as a result of any activity, incident or matter related to the occupation." It contained a dispute resolution mechanism based on the BC Labour Code and would be signed by both unions, the MHR, the Ministry of Agriculture and the BCBC.

This preliminary package of proposals grew to ten as the new management committee and union representatives prepared to meet local managers. Added to the original four proposals were a number of mechanical steps associated with de-occupation and the appointment of BCGEU and UPN members to joint working groups or committees. They also included agreement on the union and management texts of public statements on de-occupation. Most important of all was a proposal for the MHR to agree on the appointment of Vickers to the placement planning process.

On August 3, eight representatives of the union met five local management representatives. Management was represented by Terry Prysiazniuk, manager of the institution; Alex McIntosh, director of nursing; Murray Satzer, Gord Begley and Brent Johnson, personnel officers. I was the union's spokesperson with Bill Rhode, chairperson of the Kamloops local of the hospital and allied service component along with Sylvia Grant from the local; Trudy Merritt, social education and health services local; Marg Seagris, administrative services local, Brett Cornell, Component 15 BC Building Corporation, and Sam Johnson and Doris Fesser from the UPN. After I outlined the ten demands, management asked for a number of hours to consider them before reconvening.

At 3:45 p.m. the committees reconvened and management reiterated its same three points: 1. the MHR requests the union cease interference in Tranquille operations; 2. the union subscribe and adhere to existing MHR policies; and 3. the MHR would be prepared to meet with the union after the occupation ends and your submissions are received. Imagine how well that went over with the union's representatives! After two and a half weeks, we were frustrated. Needless to say, little progress was made, but the process of negotiations had started—or at least that's what we thought.

We presented a full report to the new management committee, and the bargaining committee, meeting afterwards, discussed a number of more drastic actions that would further annoy management and the ministry. No decisions were made except that I would have a quiet chat with Terry Prysiazniuk the next day: Thursday, August 4. That conversation did not go well either, and nothing was gained. The new management negotiating committee directed me to write to Prysiazniuk.

My August 4 letter to Prysiazniuk certainly showed our frustration. It stated I was writing on behalf of the committee and confirmed for him that the "abrupt departure from the afternoon meeting" (August 3) was "a direct rejection of your response." My letter demanded management alter their position that no discussions could take place until the occupation had ended. It served notice that the media blackout, which had been previously agreed upon to facilitate discussions, would end in six hours unless renewed discussions were convened. I had a long discussion with Cliff Andstein and we concluded that the MHR headquarters was in full control of the local officials and discussions at the headquarters level were needed.

In a telephone conversation with Cliff thirty-five years later, he observed to me that it was at about this time that he got the feeling that the MHR really did not want the institution back and were happy to have the workers run the place. It certainly felt that way to me as well. The August 4 minutes of the new management committee meeting featured the report of the negotiating committee. The committee focused on ways to increase pressure on old management. One of the outcomes of that discussion was the development of a directive from new management to all unionized staff at Tranquille, copied to old management. It prohibited union members from doing any work for old management including dealing with correspondence, exercising signing authority and conducting personal exchanges with old management. It further shut off phone contact to cottage F-34 where old management was huddled, and designated new management officials to carry out several joint tasks.

The next day, August 5, the back channel between MHR headquarters and BCGEU headquarters heated up immediately. The *Tough Times* reported the developments: "This evening around 7 p.m., Gary Steeves received a call from the union headquarters in Vancouver. The Ministry of Human Resources in Victoria had called headquarters to say that Mr. Prysiazniuk had a proposal to make to them as a result of new management's actions today. The union stated that all proposals would only be decided by the workers at Tranquille and there would be no deal without a written agreement stating that: a) there would be no reprisals to participants of the sit-in, and b) the unions would participate in developing a closure plan for Tranquille. After the union office passed on this message, Victoria phoned back to say that Russell Dean, personnel manager for the MHR, was ready to make a proposal in response to the ten demands of new management."

Dave McPherson and I consulted the new management committee who would make a recommendation but not a decision. The *Tough Times* reported, "A decision on the proposals will be made by the full membership of the unions at Tranquille at a meeting on Monday, August 8, 1983 at 7 p.m. in the cafeteria." Locally, the new management committee got to work on de-occupation plans including essential service staffing levels in the event of an agreement. Things were moving at lightning speed.

Cliff Andstein did a marvellous job negotiating with Russell Dean and the other MHR senior officials. Management lacked any sense of urgency and at times, Cliff's feeling that they did not want the institution back was inescapable. The next morning, Saturday, August 6, Cliff relayed a letter from Russell Dean that said the ministry would not take disciplinary action against its employees for participating in the occupation, and agreed to meet after the occupation ended to work out the rest of the details pursuant to the provisions

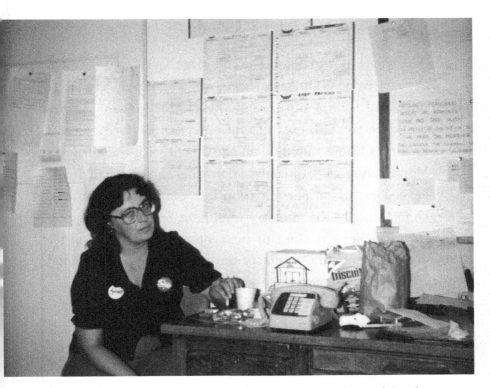

Hard-working scheduler takes a break in front of the boards containing the roster of those sitting in. Gary Steeves

of the existing collective agreement. The MHR advised Cliff that the amnesty agreement was fine, but that the parties would need to discuss other matters, including union participation in a planning committee for residents, only after the occupation had ended.

Cliff explained that the planning committee was the deal-breaker for Tranquille employees. Without a firm agreement on that matter, the employees were sure to vote "no" on any deal put to them. The collective agreement between the government and the BCGEU, which expired October 31, 1983, and Bills 2 and 3 would determine how employees would be treated, but without a say on the treatment of residents, there would be no agreement with the MHR. On Monday, August 8, Cliff advised me that the MHR had finally agreed to "union participation in a planning committee." Unfortunately, the ministry would not budge on accepting David Vickers as chair of that committee, but the other arrangements the ministry outlined were at least good enough to put to a membership vote.

The Monday night ratification meeting was tense and serious. I explained the conversations we had with Terry Prysiazniuk, the negotiating committee discussions, the strike-vote arrangements and the need to attend to preparations for collective agreement negotiations in September. I reviewed the events of Wednesday, August 3, and the union's ten-point proposal to management. I explained the Friday night call from Cliff with the MHR proposal, and I explained we had amnesty, union participation in a planning committee and a chance for further discussions with the MHR. I further explained that Cliff had told the ministry that we needed everything in writing before we could take it to our membership—and the ministry had done so!

I read the letters and recommended on behalf of the negotiating committee that we accept the MHR's offer. I then walked everyone through what our objectives had been: show our displeasure to the MHR; oppose the budget and its legislation; bring public attention to the plight of Tranquille residents; and force the government to deal with displaced workers from Tranquille. The first three had been achieved, and the fourth would be dealt with at the master bargaining negotiations between the BCGEU and the provincial government.

These negotiations covered the entire provincial public service and would deal with lay-off, recall, severance, Treasury Board Order 57 and major service terminations and institutional closures. The union had decided to take a strike vote before the collective agreement expired at midnight, October 31. I reminded members that November 1 had been set as the strike deadline as part of the Operation Solidarity strike schedule worked out by union leaders through the BC Federation of Labour. If no agreement could be reached with government, the BCGEU would be the first union to strike, taking out the entire public service. Much work needed to be done on strike arrangements, work that would be difficult to complete effectively if the occupation were still underway. Further, if the occupation agreement was accepted, we could get to work on the care plans for residents—a major achievement of the occupation and the negotiations to end it.

I concluded my remarks with a call to march out of the institution the next day, August 9, with our heads held high and continue marching to Riverside Park for the Operation Solidarity rally. All my remarks and reasoning were thoughtfully received. There was some discussion, but it was respectful and supportive. When the membership vote was taken shortly after, and once the graveyard shift had voted, 96 percent of the membership voted in favour of ending the occupation. The MHR then hand-delivered a letter to me asking the union for names so that three union nominees could be appointed to the committee managing the deinstitutionalization process.

BCGEU Vice-President Diane Wood, herself a provincial government employee who had been fired pending the passage of Bill 3, announced the de-occupation agreement to the media. The occupation would end at 2 p.m. August 9. In her public statement, Diane emphasized the agreement reached as far as the residents were concerned. Her statement said, "The agreement calls for participation by three union members on a multidisciplinary ministry planning and resource team which will plan for the future needs of residents of Tranquille who are facing relocation to the community at large." Essential service staffing levels were in place at 2 p.m. on August 9 as the workers marched out. Standards of care were maintained while everyone else joined the rally at Riverside Park. A detailed march route had been planned and the local paper later reported

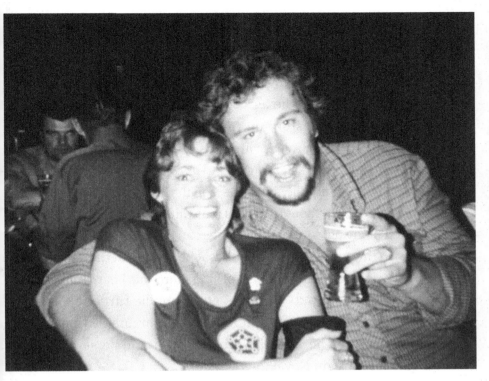

Diane Bird (Hartley) and Steve Wood at the August 9, 1983 party after occupation ended. Gary Steeves

2,500 marchers participated. Four thousand people from the Kamloops area also attended the rally. Tranquille workers received an extra-loud ovation as they entered the park.

All seemed well until the ministry issued a statement the following day concerning the end of the occupation. The statement was odd and convoluted, completely missing the spirit and intent of the de-occupation agreement. It said, "The employer does not, however, condone unauthorized absences from work and will take action against staff who take such time off for any purpose." Was Minister McCarthy trying to renege on the agreement with her officials? *The Province* carried a story on August 10 that was based on Diane Wood's news release and was headlined: "Sit-in workers escape penalty." The August 11 *Vancouver Sun* story was headlined, "Tranquille staff face penalty," and included the minister's quote about absences, but Cliff Andstein was also quoted pointing out that the minister's statement was "contrary to the agreement that was reached between the union and officials of her ministry." Nothing more was heard about discipline and BCGEU members at Tranquille turned their attention to the new planning process for institutional residents and the pending province-wide public service strike set to begin November 1.

CHAPTER ELEVEN

IT'S ABOUT THE RESIDENTS

The agreement of the MHR to allow the union into the planning process for the deinstitutionalization of Tranquille residents was a major breakthrough. It marked a huge departure from the MHR's past practices. The BCGEU had been trying for many years to influence or participate in the government's plans for a system of care for developmentally disabled people. But the government's market beliefs tended to favour contractors operating group homes as the way to go. The occupation of Tranquille had had a profound impact on the ministry's decision-makers and opened the door for the union to have a greater say in what would happen to BCGEU members and developmentally delayed residents of the three large institutions.

There were a number of reasons why the union wished to participate in shaping the future of the care system. It recognized that social change was moving people and their governments toward community living models for the developmentally disabled. The benefits of community living were well documented. Studies showed significant improvements in education and training outcomes for developmentally delayed individuals over those living in institutional circumstances. The BCGEU's hospital and allied services component (Component 2) was a large and influential segment of the union and had been a loyal and dedicated membership base in the modern history of the union. The union's engagement in public sector collective bargaining had significant support from Component 2's loyal union membership and the component maintained large locals in Victoria, the Lower Mainland and Kamloops. Change was on the horizon, and the BCGEU viewed itself as a social union well positioned to represent and protect its members in the face of that change.

Since the mid-1970s, the government of BC had a ten-year plan in place to alter the system of care for people with developmental disabilities, especially those residing in large residential schools and institutions. Financial resources did not appear to be major problems during the formative years of the ten-year plan. Government appeared to be able to afford a community care system and the cost of transitioning to it. The government was content with moving persons with developmental disabilities slowly but steadily into community-based residential care settings.

The union had strong views on the structure of the care system. For the developmentally disabled residents of the institutional schools, the structural makeup of the system needed to afford community living opportunities in group homes or similar residential living arrangements, but not small institutions. The government needed to fully fund the operation of group homes, and it must be responsible for establishing and fully funding the necessary programs and community-based services these homes would require. It was unreasonable to expect families to bear the cost of community-based services such as transportation services. Specialized transportation services were a perfect example of a community resource essential to the community living environment for deinstitutionalized residents. Unfortunately, the government's market-driven group home model pitted the care of developmentally delayed individuals against low-bid systems of choosing operators and their profit motives. Furthermore, the MHR had no standards or verification system to assess the quality of care.

The union held that the care system must have independent monitoring to oversee the operation of that system. The purpose of such monitoring would be to ensure that individual program plans with their assorted training and educational goals were being met. And further, such monitoring would act as a force to prevent neglect and abuse of developmentally delayed people. As far as the workers were concerned, the union strongly believed that part of the transition plan could include retraining and placement options for workers as well as early retirement and severance packages to enable redundant employees to leave the service if they chose to. The union insisted that large segments of experienced caregivers employed in institutional schools would be required in the new system if it were to be successful.

Nearly two years after Tranquille closed, the union's view was proven to be correct. The structural framework of a new community-based residential care model should have, in the union's opinion, been cooperatively developed by all those involved in the system. But the lack of interest shown by the MHR in discussing future plans to achieve the goals of deinstitutionalization led the union to conclude that either deinstitutionalization was not a high priority with the ministry, or the MHR was going to do it their way with little or no cooperative planning. Although the ministry had successfully closed Dellview in Vernon and divested itself of Skeenaview in Terrace, the so-called ten-year plan made little progress.

In the union's view, proper planning would increase the chances of appropriate and successful community placement for people with developmental disabilities. It would mean employment options for experienced caregivers, including Tranquille employees, and a stable transition period for Tranquille residents and the community of Kamloops. However, MHR executives, directed by Grace McCarthy and others, saw proper planning processes as an impediment to the opportunity to save money at the expense of government employees, persons with mental disabilities and the community of Kamloops.

The restraint budget of July 1983 cut funding to non-profit societies, impeding the expansion of existing group-home networks. The exception, of course, came from the secret meeting with the Kamloops Society for the Mentally Handicapped, where the ministry offered an additional $6 million to the society provided KSMH took another hundred Tranquille residents. In general, no community-based residential accommodations existed for Tranquille residents. Community-based programs and services to support Tranquille residents were not in place, as existing services were filled to capacity; therefore, no plan existed to match Tranquille residents with community residential services at levels of support they were receiving at Tranquille. No monitoring system had even been planned, let alone developed. And most fundamentally, the MHR had not developed and established standards of care for their funded agencies.

The de-occupation agreement at Tranquille resulted in the establishment of a community resources advisory committee to assess and prepare individual Tranquille residents for placement in the community. The union nominated three members to this committee. The government accepted those nominated but retained the absolute authority to appoint to the committee. At the same time, the union appointed its own internal committee made up of healthcare workers, social workers, psychiatric social workers, psychologists and nurses to monitor the placement process and provide support to the union members on the team.

As the community resources advisory committee and the other union members at Tranquille began to plan for community placement, the BCGEU mobilized for a province-wide strike set to begin on November 1, 1983. Deinstitutionalization planning, and most other activities associated with placement, slowed to a crawl as BC became preoccupied with the possibility of a general strike.

Much has been written about the massive strikes that began November 1, 1983. Newspapers at the time carried great detail about the strikes and Rod Mickleburgh's *On the Line: A History of the British Columbia Labour Movement* accurately records the steady progress toward a all-out general strike and the controversial end of strike action on November 14. Like all provincial government employees, Tranquille workers returned to work the week of November 14, after two weeks on a picket line. The BCGEU–Government of BC agreement retained the rights and protections the government had attempted to legislate away. So by early 1984, work on resident placement was well underway. Union members on the community resources advisory committee reported progress in the fight for suitable placements.

Discontent, however, was growing with the push by management to meet Grace McCarthy's December 31, 1984 closure deadline. Field workers reported similar pressure

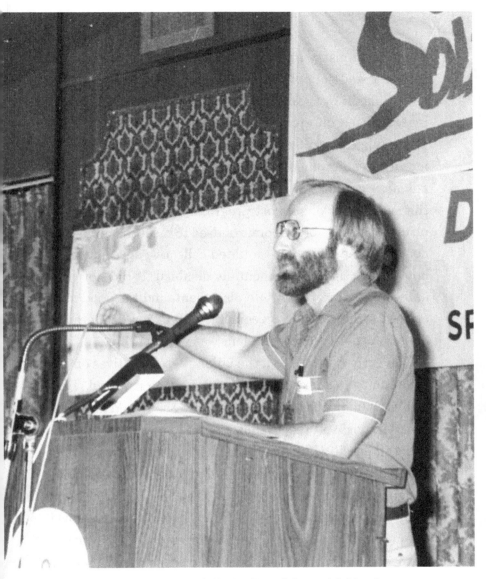

Cliff Andstein, director of the Collective Bargaining and Arbitration
department of the BCGEU. BCGEU Archives

from the ministry as they attempted to arrange community living and support services. Their jobs were becoming more difficult by the day. Internal union discussions increasingly focused on growing evidence that the MHR wanted Tranquille closed at any cost but on schedule. In the opinion of the union members from the community resources advisory committee, the quality of community services, the availability of support programs and the adequacy of placements were being compromised to meet the ministry's deadline. The recently negotiated collective agreement did not protect the developmentally disabled. It did not guarantee proper or appropriate placement, and the good faith of the de-occupation agreement calling for cooperative development of placement plans was wearing thin.

In early April of 1984, the union representatives on the community resources advisory committee revolted. They met with union officials and announced they could no longer sanction nor lend their reputation to the placement plans being imposed by management. For example, residents of Tranquille who were enrolled in day programs were being assigned to group homes in communities where no such program existed. Some hastily established homes did not meet Community Care Licensing Act requirements. For a variety of reasons, other group homes were considered inappropriate for the placement of residents, and forty or fifty residents were rumoured to be headed for long-term care facilities. The community resources advisory committee said the easy placements were complete and the most difficult placements were not being properly arranged. They advised union officials that funding quarrels between the MHR and non-profit societies and lack of support services in ill-prepared communities jeopardized chances of success for many developmentally delayed Tranquille residents.

In light of the limited ability of the union to influence the MHR's policy and planning processes regarding deinstitutionalization, the union was faced with two choices. It could allow the MHR's flawed policies and procedures to develop a care system for which the government is only marginally responsible and rely on the collective agreement to protect institutional workers, or the union could press its case for a community care system for which the government is directly responsible and accountable. The latter system would provide better quality of care for the intellectually challenged, and better working environments and job security for those workers experienced in the care of persons with intellectual disabilities. Local union representatives and President Richards on behalf of the provincial executive agreed that a plan of action must be developed. The union members of the community resources advisory committee agreed to stay on the ministry's planning team and fight for better decisions.

At a union meeting of Tranquille members on April 11, 1984, a plan of action was proposed and enthusiastically endorsed by the membership. It called for the launching of

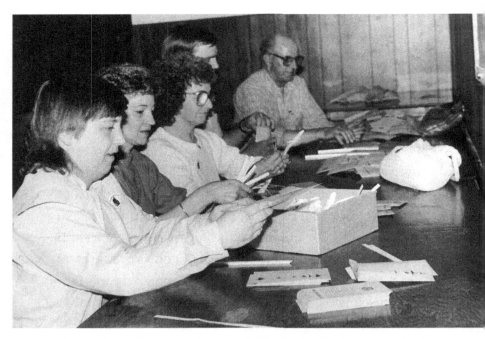

Tranquille members preparing material for the Quality Care Campaign in 1984. BCGEU Archives

a community campaign to deal with the impact of the MHR policies on the developmentally disabled and the community at large. The union had come full circle in its involvement in the issue of deinstitutionalization. From the outrage felt by union leaders and members at the potential treatment of developmentally delayed persons and employees, to the satisfaction of being invited to participate in the development of a care system, to the disappointment of the bureaucratic and political expediency exhibited by the MHR officials, the union had tried every tactic at its disposal to achieve effective social reform. Unions are sometimes considered organizations that simply protect their own interests, but the Tranquille case is a great demonstration of a union being more than altruistic.

During the occupation, for example, BCGEU representatives and local officers stood up to a neighbourhood group who opposed the establishment of a group home in their neighbourhood. One homeowner remarked during the meeting, "But you guys are supposed to be opposed to the closure." The BCGEU was not opposed to deinstitutionalization; the BCGEU was opposed to residents being taken for granted and treated like a burden on the public purse rather than as important members of our communities. The BCGEU stood for social justice, efficient public services and fair treatment for all. The de-occupation agreement resulted in an agreement that allowed the union to have a role in planning for community placement and the closure of an institution. The continued efforts of the MHR to meet artificial deadlines proved David Vickers to be deadly accurate in his initial assessment and fears of the MHR's closure plans. The BCGEU and its members in the MHR, especially those at Tranquille, had done their best to raise the issues and create a climate for change.

On December 31, 1984, the Tranquille school closed, in keeping with the Ministry of Human Resources' self-imposed deadline. The MHR met its deadline, but did not exert its best efforts for every resident. It was only possible to meet the deadline through the provincial cabinet authorizing the abandonment of deinstitutionalization for fifty-four Tranquille residents, transferring them to the Glendale institution in Victoria. David Vickers' original pronouncement was extremely accurate; when one is dealing with human beings, hard deadlines just don't work. If one is committed to deinstitutionalization and community care, the development of community resources and amenities must be pursued with no artificial deadlines.

The Kamloops Society for the Mentally Handicapped accommodated the largest group of former Tranquille residents, but community placement of residents occurred throughout other areas of BC, too. Success varied, but the union members on the community resources advisory committee did the best they could in spite of the ministry's haste. The committee worked hard to ensure placements were appropriate for the former residents, but was disbanded when the last fifty-four residents were transferred. The union's committee to support the community resources advisory committee members was also disbanded after the institution closed.

Collectively, the committee members felt they had done all they could given the difficult circumstances imposed by the MHR. As I told the *Vancouver Sun* on July 29, "It has been agreed with management since this thing started that the care and comfort of the residents are paramount. That's what it is all about in the first place." The union had stayed true to its intentions and done all it could to assist residents and their families with a transition that was hurried by the ministry and underfunded by the government.

A July 31 letter to the editor of the *Kamloops Daily Sentinel* from Leslie Payne, a healthcare worker at Tranquille, asked the right question based on the facts at Tranquille. She described programs and services available to residents including picnics; camping trips to Pine Park, Camp Winfield, Shuswap Lake and Vancouver; swimming at the YMCA pool, the Westsyde Pool or their own Tranquille pool; movies at the recreation hall; live entertainment on special occasions like Christmas and Valentine's Day; home-living, pre-vocational, handicraft, carpentry and communications skills; attending hockey games, rodeos and circuses; and recreation outings to go roller skating and bowling. She noted the respite care Tranquille provided for families and group-home operators and cited the multidisciplinary team of social workers, psychologists, doctors, nurses, health-care workers and volunteers who worked together at the institution for the good of residents. She asked, "Will these residents have the same opportunities in the community?" The truth, of course, was that some residents were better off after the closure, but others were not. Only community resources advisory committee professionals and residents and their families could judge for certain, but from my observations and involvement, the government failed too many families and residents.

Very few of the public statements by cabinet ministers turned out to be true. Attorney General Brian Smith, for example, told the Victoria bureau of the *Vancouver Sun* that the government was "reconsidering its method of implementing restraint measures." There is no evidence in cabinet documents and records of any reconsideration discussions ever taking place, nor were there records of decisions of any reconsiderations taking place. In fact, there is evidence to the contrary, as the premier insisted on the discipline of his ministers to restrict activities and statements concerning the 1983 budget and its accompanying legislation. Clearly, the premier did not want to fuel expectations that could be used to attack the government's position.

The November 1983 Operation Solidarity strikes included the BCGEU strike against the government and collective agreement negotiations succeeded in keeping the contractual protections of the expiring agreement. Tranquille employees retained the protections, rights and options they fought for since the beginning of the occupation. For BCGEU members, Bills 2 and 3 were defeated. In fact, BCGEU negotiators had improved the rights and options available to displaced workers covered by the BCGEU master and component collective agreements between the government of BC and the BCGEU. Some Tranquille workers retired with enhanced pension entitlements while others took severance and went to work outside the public sector as caregivers in non-profit societies' group homes such as the Kamloops

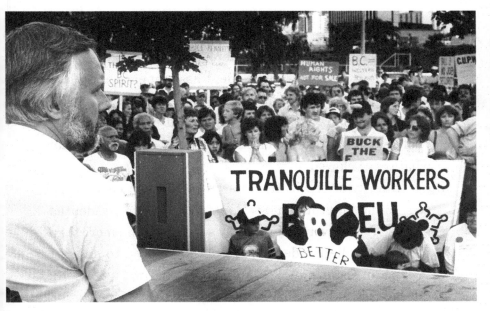

Tranquille workers protest in front of Kamloops MLA Claude Richmond.

BCGEU Archives

Society. Many Tranquille workers took alternate employment in the public sector, either in the Kamloops area or by transferring to the MHR facilities at Woodlands in New Westminster and Glendale in Victoria. In general, Treasury Board Order 57 provisions and the revised collective agreements cushioned Tranquille workers, but forced many employees to leave the Kamloops area.

Were the union's efforts to change government policy worth it? Was the occupation, the de-occupation agreement, and the community resources advisory committee and support efforts worth it? I think the answer is yes. So many residential placements were improved because of the work of our members on resident assessments and placement planning. So many residents experienced better deinstitutionalization outcomes than if the workers, the professionals or the union members had not stood up for what they believed in.

Deinstitutionalization, however, had serious deficiencies. Many institutional residents ended up in residential situations that were not properly supported, and more than fifty Tranquille residents were merely moved to another institution. Cabinet records show that in the mid-1980s, MHR officials knew they could not achieve deinstitutionalization for all Tranquille residents. But the union had run a successful community campaign advocating for quality care for the developmentally disabled, and lived to fight another day. Over the succeeding years, the BCGEU organized thousands of care workers looking for effective and socially progressive union representation. These workers were employed by group-home operators and became major players in the community social services sector of the provincial economy. And crucially, the residents were certainly better off for the efforts of the union.

EPILOGUE

W hat is it, thirty-five years or more later, that we can learn from the occupation of Tranquille? First, workers and I would say citizens in general have an inherent sense of social justice. They know right from wrong and, if given the chance, will act to create higher and better outcomes on social issues. In the case of Tranquille, however, the workers were not only well-tuned to right and wrong, they were incredibly brave and strong in carrying out actions to support their beliefs. Second, elections really do matter. Polling before the 1983 election showed Dave Barrett and his New Democrats with a slight lead and some real possibility of forming a government in 1983.

The public mood changed when Barrett made some negative remarks about the Social Credit's restraint program, particularly its compensation stabilization program. It seems that restricting government employees' wage increases resonated with the 20 percent of the BC workforce who were unemployed. Rather than consider which party can get those people back to work, people resented others getting help while they struggled. The public mood shifted, and Bill Bennett won a majority in the BC legislature. Bennett and his Social Credit gang seriously misled British Columbians. The whole restraint thing was a lie. People were hurting and needed help, but the Socreds lied about their budget being balanced. Later, they said it was just a slight $800 million miscalculation. The opposition revealed the fraud after the election, but people had bought the line that restraint, a balanced budget and Social Credit leadership would get them the help they sought.

As insiders concede, Bennett and the other leaders of the Social Credit administration had decided to get rid of their political opposition in 1983, or at least damage them extensively. Cabinet staffers made no bones about describing the disdain with which Social Credit staff and elected representatives held for NDPers generally and the BCGEU in particular. Social Credit decided to gut the civil service, eliminate the Rentalsman Office, wipe out the Human Rights Commission, stifle or eliminate bona fide collective bargaining and labour standards as found in the Employment Standards Act, the Labour Code of BC and the Public Service Labour Relations Act. They embarked on their dark agenda because they believed it would reduce the size of government and cripple their opposition. The Social Credit's philosophical belief in letting the market decide was only cheap political rhetoric. The desire to rid themselves of their political opposition and the tools their opponents used to fight for a civil society required legislative intervention, not Adam Smith's invisible hand. The widespread attack on civil society launched by the Socreds in 1983 was prompted by the desire for political control, not just economic reform. In the minds of some cabinet insiders, political control trumped the economic game plan of Bennett's government. In hindsight, the Social Credit legislative attack only motivated unions and a large cross-section of British Columbians to tell the government they were wrong.

Bennett went too far in his budget cuts and program eliminations. Poking his finger in the eye of every middle-income taxpayer simply backfired. His personal approval rating fell well below that of his party's support, he failed to achieve the Bill 2 and 3 restrictions on public sector unions and he resigned as premier before the end of his term of office. Bennett had stubbornly refused to take one of his father's famous second looks when he tried to continue his program of budget cuts and restraint.

When he cut funding to residential living opportunities such as small group homes and community-based support programs for the developmentally disabled, he aggravated natural allies who quickly found the BCGEU to be a more reasonable and progressive ally. Advocacy groups for the developmentally disabled had mistrusted the BCGEU, but Bill Bennett left the advocates high and dry in the political arena. The advocacy organizations, notwithstanding David Vickers' warnings, had relied on government promises made by Premier Bennett which turned out to be outright falsehoods. Budget savings from government staffing cuts such as Tranquille went to the mining and forest industries through such mechanisms as Vote 40.

Electing more trustworthy leaders would have made a big difference. It really does matter who we elect, but unfortunately making those determinations is never easy and is sometimes very difficult. One can understand how deinstitutionalization advocates got sucked in by the promises to act on something they felt very strongly about. Tranquille shows us that politics and elections do matter. These events emphasize how important informed citizens are, and how essential it is to have trustworthy elected officials. Elections are about people. In my opinion, we must find leaders with love, kindness and compassion in their hearts as opposed to those who feel their mission is to represent and protect business interests at all costs. When we are choosing who best to lead our government, erring on the side of humanity is our wisest choice. Civil society depends on it. And elections really do matter.

What other lessons might we learn from Tranquille? Another observation from the thirty-five-year-old events of Tranquille is that unions are very important participants in a civil society. Without the BCGEU, the government of BC would have encountered fewer obstacles to their original

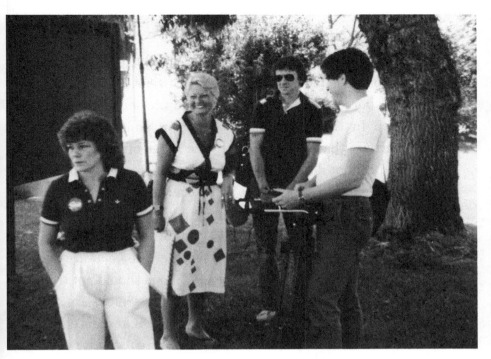

Second Vice-President Diane Wood with media at Tranquille, August 1983.

BCGEU Archives

plans for Tranquille and the province. Without a healthy labour movement in general, the government would have encountered few, if any, organizations in the province with the resources and expertise to force the government to rethink its legislative agenda. A future civil society very much depends on a healthy, democratic union movement. Unions have social obligations as well as obligations to their own members. It is this social obligation that the rank-and-file members at Tranquille understood so well. They believed in a civil society and were prepared to accept it as a social obligation—as union members and as citizens.

My personal observations, based on being directly involved in the Tranquille occupation and Operation Solidarity, is that unions have a wide range of things they can and cannot do. They can campaign to change people's minds, express their opinions, and influence decisions. They can negotiate solutions to complex problems, create better problem-solving processes and achieve better outcomes for ordinary citizens. Unions, however, need to be aware of things they would be better to avoid. Unions should not try to dictate, and they should never go it alone. Unions are at their best when they engage in conversation and develop strong allies to their cause. Union power is real, but it does not need to be lorded over anyone to be effective. Some people have said, "Well the institution closed so what was the point?" To them I point out that the time for deinstitutionalization had arrived, and Tranquille was to be reduced in scope and eventually closed one way or the other. The BCGEU just tried to make them do it in a more sensitive and compassionate way for all involved. And I think we succeeded.

From the traditional union perspective, a union cannot refuse to respond when an employer says they are going to terminate six hundred employees and eliminate any rights those employees may have had in that process. When employers abandon any and all concerns for their employees, unions must act. It delivers the wrong message to any employer for unions to be inactive when their members are threatened. Unions have, as the member in the back of the cafeteria said, no choice but to act. The union was responsible for attempting to ensure residents were placed in good community settings, or better community situations than would have otherwise been the case. The union used its bargaining power and its members' expertise to force itself into the transition process. If there had not been an occupation, there would not have been a de-occupation agreement with a community resource advisory committee and union involvement.

The Tranquille occupation proved to me that unions could affect the policy of government and act as a societal conscience in the face of regressive governments. Unions can use collective bargaining processes to effect outcomes for the community at large. Although unions have not routinely taken actions that bring community and social issues to the bargaining table, it is time to consider doing so more often. In some cases, unions have adopted a social policy stance, avoiding the temptation to stick to bread-and-butter issues, but social unionism on a wider and more profound scale is entirely possible and definitely necessary. In the twenty-first century, social unionism must replace bread-and-butter unionism and put both the economic and social issues of its members and their families on the bargaining table. Unions must strive to deliver benefits for union members, their families, their communities and the planet Mother Earth provides for us.

I could not conclude any retrospective of the Tranquille story without recognizing the bravery, fearlessness and determination of the employees of that institution. Thirty-five years later, I can only marvel at how superb Tranquille's employees were in virtually everything they did. The MHR looked for any reason or critical point to discredit their workers or have them arrested. They could find nothing as far as care of residents and safety of those in care was concerned. Members of both the BCGEU and the UPN were outstanding in how they conducted themselves during the occupation and after its conclusion. The workers knew the world was watching and they performed superbly, improving care and related services, providing better attention to the physical plant and equipment, and showing just how good they were at running the institution.

Later in the occupation, in an interview with one of the newspapers, old management head Terry Prysiazniuk said the conditions under the occupation were very safe and comfortable for residents, their families and other visitors. In fact, union representatives on the community resources advisory committee later told me that the number of incidents of problematic behaviour with residents during the occupation was significantly lower than comparable three-week periods. Perhaps this can be explained by a letter from Tony Gusman to the editor of the *Kamloops News* dated

August 10 in which he said, "The sit-in has in many ways proved to be exemplary exercise in cooperation, mutual support, and an extraordinary human experience for the participants."

BCGEU and UPN members were simply selfless in their relationships with residents, their families and the public. I don't think old management ever realized how fortunate they were to have a group of such dedicated people working in their institution. The workers' loyalty to their union was second only to their loyalty to the residents they cared for. I arrived at Tranquille in the middle of the night, made suggestions, issued directives and took over a variety of functions. No one questioned Dave McPherson or me other than to ensure residents came first and we had the information we needed to help lead their protest.

Two weeks into the occupation, a *Tranquille Tough Times* reporter asked me, tongue-in-cheek, "After following you blindly for fourteen days, we would like to know how long you have been with the union?" Tranquille employees understood they were the union and they effectively engaged in a grassroots form of democracy that most people could only dream of in their communities. They met nightly, made decisions and elected their leaders. They directed union staff like Dave and me and ran a large institution flawlessly. And they did so with expertise, compassion and love. I spoke on their behalf in an August 9 *Kamloops News* interview, observing, "We changed priorities. In a microcosm where people can't take care of themselves, a more loving and caring approach to our world is needed."

One example of the efficiency of Tranquille union members and activists was the management of their own communications committee. The committee did everything to keep everyone informed without fanfare or handholding. They were like pros, but none actually were. They wrote logical letters and they wrote emotional letters. They expressed collective wisdom and frustration. They published a daily info sheet, the *Tough Times*, which was to the point yet informative, serious yet light-hearted. When I reread every issue in my research for this book, I was amazed at how on point and informative they were each and every day.

While Tranquille taught me that unions can effect public policy, it showed me that it takes focus, energy and discipline to do so. I told the *Kamloops Daily Sentinel* during the August 9 de-occupation that "what we have proven at Tranquille is you can fight the government without hurting those who need your services." The BCGEU always negotiated essential service levels before any dispute or work stoppage in the government service. In many ways, the BCGEU was a leader in how to responsibly exercise its right to strike.

Tranquille also taught me not to take the union's power and ability to do big things for granted. Unions are collections of humans who have pooled their resources to be either a simple insurance policy or a mobilized army or something in between. A union should always be focused on the greater good and that good is a truly democratic society. Employers' rights are fundamentally anti-democratic and make workplaces more hostile and less productive. Unions should use their power to challenge, every day, the employers' rights to dictate to their employees. Unions must expand the role and responsibility of workers to run society in a more wise and caring manner. They must defy the mean-spirited bean-counters!

And that is what the new management committee did as their last act upon de-occupation. They issued a one-page list of *do*s and *don't*s. It started with the statement that "following the ending of the occupation, it is important that all local officers, stewards and members recognize the rights and protections which are provided due to union membership and the collective agreement." It listed four *don't*s and seven *do*s and concluded with, "Remember you should be putting management in the situation of not second-guessing your abilities as a worker in advance of the work being done."

Tranquille showed me that workers can do just about anything they put their minds to. Workers don't need someone leaning over their shoulder, second-guessing their methods or intentions. Workers don't need bosses that have never done the work themselves trying to tell the worker what to do or how to do it. Well-trained workers are worth their weight in gold, and Tranquille had a full cast of well-trained workers.

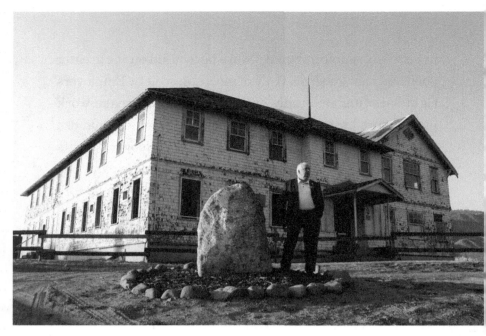

Darryl Walker, BCGEU president 2008–2014, on a visit to Tranquille.

BCGEU Archives

Finally, a note about the BCGEU. Through the 1980s, the BCGEU proved time and again they were not a business union but were very much a social union. The BCGEU was keenly aware of and prepared to act on social issues. Whether on their own or through the BC Federation of Labour, the Canadian Labour Congress or local labour councils, the BCGEU was out front on a wide variety of social issues. A scan of BCGEU convention resolutions will reinforce the notion of the BCGEU being socially conscious and a social policy advocate.

The BCGEU also became an organizing union. It started immediately after the battles of 1983 and intensified during Bill Vander Zalm's tenure as premier. It came into full bloom in the 1990s with changes to the labour code as the union responded to large numbers of workers wanting union representation. Two years in a row in the nineties, the BCGEU organized over five thousand new members annually. It expanded its components, diversified its occupational groups and made the BCGEU bigger and stronger. This organizing success was due in some measure to the organization of groups like non-profit group home workers and for-profit home support workers. Care workers flocked to the BCGEU, and I believe it was due in part to the union's reputation and ability to represent workers and advocate for the vulnerable. Today, the BCGEU continues to be an intelligently led, socially progressive and seriously democratic union devoted to its members and the important work those members do. BC is lucky to have it.

ACKNOWLEDGEMENTS

This project would never have happened if not for the encouragement of Labour Heritage Centre past-president Ken Novakowski and executive director Donna Sacuta, the advice of my dear friend Keith Reynolds guiding me through the FOI-request maze, and Cliff Andstein urging me to write for thirty-four years.

I could not tell the story without access to facts from both sides of the story. The BCGEU archives found my daily binder of meeting notes, to-do lists and press releases, as well as a couple of boxes of other materials from the occupation. My FOI request for cabinet and other government documents led me to the BC Public Archives and a research agreement that gave me unrestricted access to all provincial cabinet minutes and documents from November 1982 until December 1986. Together with my interviews of former cabinet members and staff, I was able to establish the story from both sides of the political fence. I simply cannot thank enough the BC Archives staff for their assistance and professionalism.

For an extensive profile and description of Tranquille's buildings and lands see Gena Crowston's excellent book, *The Ghosts of Tranquille Past.*

Tranquility Lost would not have been possible without the active participation of the BCGEU. Stephanie Smith, Paul Finch, Kari Michaels, Gerri Inaba, Brian Gardiner, Diane Wood and many others helped in ways big and small. All of them have been so competent and helpful.

Others were essential to the full story. Debbie Patten, Gordon Hanson, Sheila Malcolmson and Marguerite Jackson were generous, helpful and supportive.

I was given the facts, documents and opinions of those involved but any mistake in the text is mine and mine alone. I am truly grateful to everyone involved including Howard and Silas White and their staffs at Harbour Publishing and Nightwood Editions.

INDEX

Adams, Jack, 30, 48, 49, 50, 51, 75, 96, 98, 100, 103

Andstein, Cliff, XI–XIV, 35, 48, 49, 157–59, 160, 164–68, 172, 179

Arnould, Janet, 122, 156

Barber, Charles, 35, 36

Barrett, Dave, 10–11, 34–35, 36–37, 39, 189–90

Bawlf, Sam, 35–36

BC Association of Social Workers (BCASW), III

BC Building Corporation (BCBC), 32, 121, 124, 125, 128, 130–35, 161–62

BC Chamber of Commerce, 17

BC Federation of Labour, XI–XII, 30–31, 50, 95–96, 141, 156–57, 169

Begley, Gord, 159, 163

Bennett, Bill, IX, 2, 11–14, 20–21, 22, 23–24, 70–71, 74, 94, 149, 150–52, 190–92

Bennett, W.A.C., 5–10, 20, 63–65

Bills 2 and 3, 17–18, 27–31, 32–33, 47–48, 72, 92–94, 155, 157, 160, 168, 170, 186, 191

Bird, Diane, 100–2, 171

Blencoe, Robin, 36
Boechler, Dave, 122
British Columbia
    Association for the
    Mentally Retarded
    (BCAMR), 70–71, 110–11,
    112–13
Brookes, Dawn, 122, 156
Brown, Archie, 122
Bruner, Linda, 122
Butler, Dick, 42

Canadian Labour Congress,
    96–97, 200
cerebral palsy, 64, 132
Clark, Elise, 70–71, 112–13
Community Involvement
    Program (CIP), 111
community resources
    advisory committee,
    177–81, 184, 185, 187,
    196
Copeland, Joch, 122
Cornell, Brett, 163
Cownden, Maurice, 135
Curtis, Hugh, XI, 22–27, 32

Dean, Russell, 42, 47, 92,
    166–67
Dellview (Vernon), 4, 62,
    176
Dermody, Wayne, 50–51

Employment Standards
    Act, 17–18, 30, 190

Fesser, Doris, 122, 163
Forehead, Debbie, 138–42
Freebury, Kathe, 122
Fryer, John, 50, 53, 96–97,
    109, 158–59

Gabelmann, Colin, 39
Gaglardi, Phil, 63–65
Gardom, Garde, 14
Gibson, Gordon, 12
Glendale Lodge, 57, 61,
    125–26, 183–84, 187
Grant, Sylvia, 163
Green, Terry, 121
group homes, 110–11, 117,
    118, 173, 174–75, 177,
    180, 183, 185, 186–88,
    191, 201

Gusman, Tony, 196–97

Hales, Dan, 159
Hall, Ernie, 35
Hanson, Gordon, 34, 38
Holtby, Mark, 34
Howard, Frank, 36

Iacobucci, Angelo, 89–90
Ireland, Erin, 110, 116–17, 122

Johnson, Brent, 159, 163
Johnson, John, 116–17
Johnson, Sam, 163

Kamloops Society for the Mentally Handicapped (KSMH), 65, 110–11, 113, 114, 117–18, 184
Kelly, Isabel A., 18–19
King, Bill, 38–39

Lalonde, Bob, 122
Lowndes, Al, 51–52

MacArthur, Ian, 122
Macdonald, Alex, 36
MacKinnon, Dave, 137, 153
Mahoney, Bill, 97
McCarthy, Grace, 1, 2, 69, 84–85, 91, 93, 105, 116, 117, 136, 141, 147–49, 159, 171–72, 176–77, 178
McIntosh, Alex, 66, 116, 126, 159, 163
McPherson, Dave, 51, 52–54, 75, 78–80, 82–83, 100, 117, 121, 134, 138, 159, 161–62, 166, 197
Meakes, Dan, 117
Meggs, Geoff, 10
Merrit, Trudy, 163
Mickleburgh, Rod, 10, 178

National Institute on Retardation, 110–11, 114
National Union of Provincial Government Employees, 109

neoliberalism, XI, 13–14,
  16–17, 20, 23–24,
  190–191
New Democratic Party
  (NDP), 7–8, 9, 10–11, 13,
  32–39, 108, 155, 189,
  190
Noble, John, 42, 84, 90–91,
  92, 157–58, 159–60

Operation Solidarity, 28,
  30, 38, 140, 161, 169–70,
  186, 194

Patten, Debbie. See
  Forehead, Debbie
Payne, Leslie, 185
Pearson Hospital, 62
Piper, Terry, 42
Plecas, Bob, 98, 103
Prysiazniuk, Terry, 85–86,
  133–135, 159, 163–65,
  168, 196
Purvey, Diane, 65

Rhode, Bill, 53–55, 84, 115,
  163
Richards, Norm, 84, 90–91,
  92–93, 96–97, 109, 126,
  157, 159–60, 181
Riis, Nelson, 107–9
Riverview Hospital, 57, 61
Robinson, Robbie, 76–77,
  96–100, 102–3
Royal Canadian Mounted
  Police (RCMP), 76–77,
  94–103
Russell, Bill, 122

Satzer, Murray, 163
Seagris, Marg, 122, 163
Shields, John, 18
Shtokalko, Pat, 122
Skeenaview Lodge
  (Terrace)4, 62, 72, 176
Skelly, Bob, 109
Smith, Brian, 186
Social Credit Party, 1–2,
  4–9, 11–18, 20–40,
  63–65, 70–74, 90,
  94, 102–103, 143, 155,
  190–191

Spector, Norman, 98, 103
Stupich, Dave, 25–27, 36

Tranquille Tough Times,
    89, 142–152, 165–166,
    197–198
tuberculosis, 2, 57, 59, 63

Union of Psychiatric
    Nurses (UPN)107, 112–
    113, 120–121, 124, 146,
    162–163, 196–197

Vander Zalm, Bill, 201
Vickers, David, 39, 111–114,
    118, 162–163, 168, 183–
    184, 192

Wallace, Lawrie, 35
Wood, Diane, 18, 170, 172,
    193
Wood, Steve, 100–102, 121,
    127, 159, 171
Woodlands School, 57,
    60–61, 64–66, 104, 126,
    187

Young, Phyllis, 34

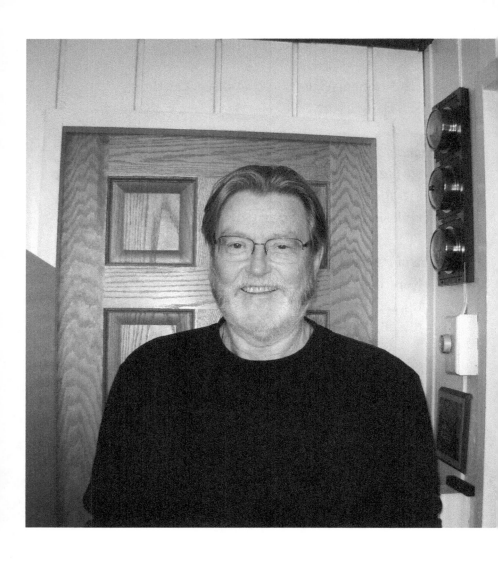

ABOUT THE AUTHOR

Gary Steeves has worked for social and environmental justice all his adult life. A staff representative with the BCGEU from 1979 to 2004, he served as director of the union from 1993 to 2004. He also served on numerous government boards and agencies, including the BC Labour Force Development Board and the Industry Training and Apprenticeship Commission, and held various positions in the union movement, including executive council member of the BC Federation of Labour. From 2004 to 2014, he served on the Islands Trust Council, including six years as vice-chair.